BodyWise

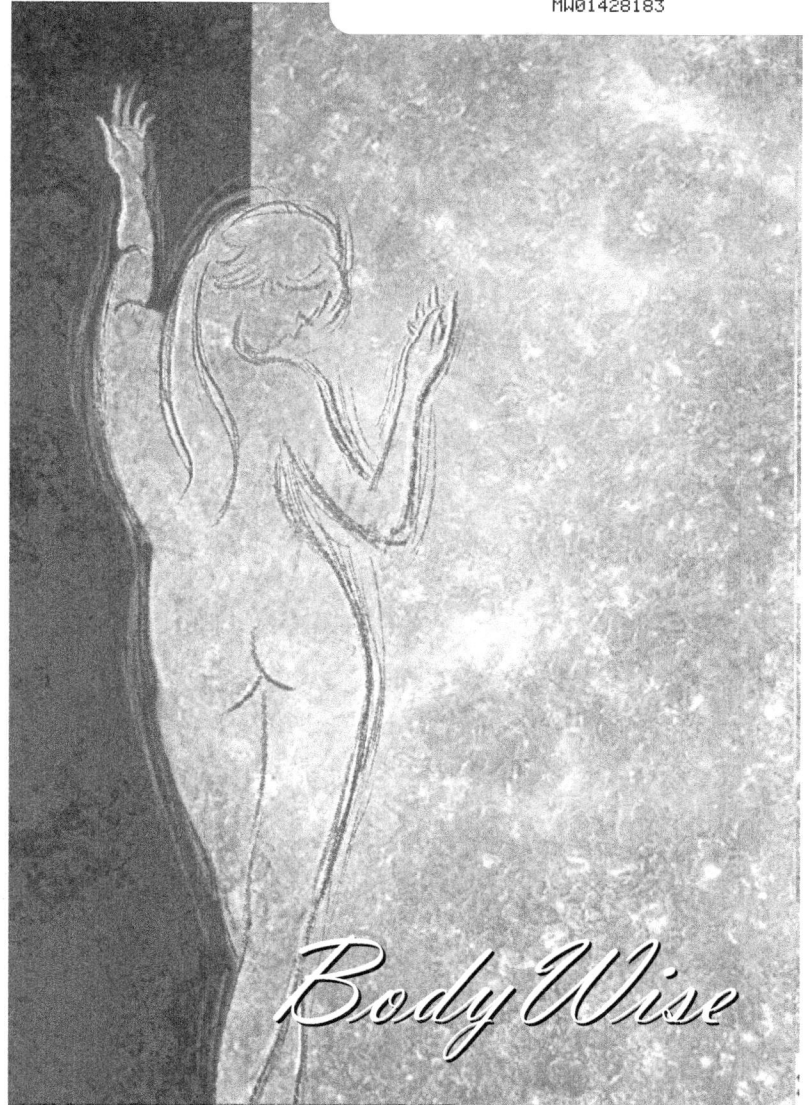

Ara Wiseman examines the health factors behind a beauty topic that affects nearly all women of all sizes. She weaves the journey of her own food education to describe how a wide range of elements contribute to the formation and clearance of cellulite. In guiding us to reach for, and to steer clear of particular foods, she delves expertly through a range of factors from the importance of food chemistry, to detoxification, stress and hydration. Wiseman teaches the why behind each lifestyle tip she offers. Beyond the classic "you are what you eat," this is a positive and empowering guide to building resilient health and beauty from the inside out.

~ Dr. Allison Freeman, Naturopathic Doctor

— • —

I have known Ara for almost 20 years, having worked with her as a teenager and again in my adult life. She has guided me in my transition from an animal based diet to healthful plant based diet with ease. I have never felt more in tune with my inner being, and it is largely thanks to Ara for her infinite wisdom and her reminder that the most important act of all is to be kind and forgiving to myself and to nourish my body with love.

~ Kerri Mozessohn

— • —

Ara has a very calming nature to her. Her spiritual energy sets a tone of ease and complete serenity. What makes Ara so special is her ability to teach us not only how to feed our bodies, but how to feed our souls as well. She sets the groundwork to start rebuilding and transforming our relationships with food.

~ Natalie Schinke

Over the past eight years I've worked with Ara on several books. I was delighted to learn that it's never too late to experience the huge benefits of changing how you eat; your body is very forgiving and will bounce back. In this new book, that same wisdom applies as Ara shows you how to take charge of diminishing that dreaded cellulite at the cellular level. Read this book – and become empowered with the awareness that *yes you can* make those changes. And it's YOU that will reap the rewards.

~ *Janet Matthews, Co-author of* Chicken Soup for the Canadian Soul

— • —

Ara has been and continues to be an excellent resource for expert knowledge, guidance and support in seeking a total healthy lifestyle including nutrition, wellness, emotional balance and dealing with stress. Her positivity, support and guidance have been a strong source of support for me over the years.

~ *Lyle Goodis*

— • —

I met Ara Wiseman in 2008 when I attended one of her presentations at my former gym. That's how our relationship began. I felt a connection with Ara and that she cared. I was at a point in my life where I was having many digestive issues and the cause was unknown. Ara helped me with a regime and I started to eat better. Ara is someone I turn to, to get me back on track. She has a deep passion and belief for what she does.

~ *Holly Neil*

A Smoother You

A Smoother You

Cellulite Secrets Revealed

Ara Wiseman, RHN, ROHP, RNCP

Maiden Tree Media
2016

Body Awareness Books:
A Smoother You : Cellulite Secrets Revealed
©2016 Ara Wiseman

All rights reserved. No part of this publication may be reproduced or transmitted in any form or by any means, electronic or mechanical, including photocopying, recording, or any information storage and retrieval system, without the prior written consent of the writer or publisher, except in the case of brief excerpts in critical reviews and articles. All inquiries should be addressed to:

Maiden Tree Media,
109 Everden Road, Toronto, Ontario M6C 3K7

www.arawiseman.com
E-mail: info@arawiseman.com

ISBN 978-0-9866090-1-5

Cataloguing data available from Library and Archives Canada

The entire contents of this book are provided for informational purposes only. No part whatsoever is intended as medical advice or as a substitute for medical or other health advice. You should always consult with a medical doctor or other health care practitioner before taking any dietary, nutritional, herbal or homeopathic supplements or beginning or stopping any therapy. Readers should use their own judgment or consult with a physician or holistic health expert for specific applications to their individual problems.

When changing your diet, there is always some reaction. Consequently, neither the author the publisher nor any party responsible for the production of this book is responsible for any adverse detoxification reactions or consequences of any kind whatsoever resulting from any information or suggestions including product suggestions, recommendations or procedures described herein. The author has attempted to provide an understanding of the topics discussed and to ensure accuracy; however, the author and all parties associated with the production of this book assume no responsibility for errors, inaccuracies, omission, or any inconsistencies herein.

Editorial: Ian Korman *&* Avia Wiseman
Cover/interior design: Intuitive Design International Ltd.
Interior image: Gary Wein

Dedication

I dedicate this book to my beautiful daughter Avia, who has taught me unconditional love, compassion, gratitude, patience, faith, and of course, fashion. I am so proud of you, you are in my heart and I love you deeply. May your life be an inspiration for others.

To my mom Boycie, who is always there for me no matter what. I love you with all my heart. To my father, Foiky and Oth Moth, DeAnn thank you for all your love and support. To my brother Jay for reminding me to keep my heart open and to Kimmy for helping me formulate the beginning of this book.

To my partner Ian, for your love, friendship, and humor, and always being there for me with all my crazy deadlines. I love you and thank you for coming into my life.

And to Karen Thomas for being my right hand and friend and for helping to intuitively design this book!

Contents

	Introduction	9
	How to Use This Book	13
1.	The Importance of Hydration	15
2.	Free Radical Damage: How It Contributes to Cellulite	18
3.	Collagen, Elastin and Strong Connective Tissues	27
4.	How Much Body Fat Should I Have?	38
5.	How to Reduce Excess Fat	47
6.	How Acid Contributes to Excess Body Fat	57
7.	Insulin and Body Fat Regulation	66
8.	Healthy Blood Vessels	70
9.	Maintaining Healthy Cell Membranes	75
10.	The Hormone Connection	80
11.	Detoxification and Its Positive Effects	88
12.	The Detoxification Process	93
13.	Your Daily Detoxification Routine	99
14.	Exercise and the Lymphatic System	103
15.	Yoga Routines for Cellulite Reduction	107

Contents (cont'd)

16. Exercises for Cellulite Reduction 118
17. Meal Planning Guide for Cellulite Reduction 125
18. Recipes 131
19. Tidbits to Chew On 167
20. Charts :
    Dirty Dozen™ / Clean 15™ 170
    Protein Charts 171

Footnotes 173
References 174

Introduction

Whether or not you currently have cellulite, at some point in your life you will look in the mirror and see dimpled flesh starring back at you. It doesn't matter whether you are thin, athletic, need to lose a few pounds, or even more than a few pounds—cellulite does not discriminate.

In my nutritional counseling practice, I teach clients how to get rid of the bumpy, lumpy skin on their arms, buttocks, and thighs. Most people are surprised to discover that through proper nutrition they can become healthier, slow down the aging of their skin, as well as drastically diminish their cellulite.

The pursuit of optimal health has always been a journey and an ongoing evolution for me. I've been interested in and have studied nutrition my entire life. Nutrition is my passion, and I'm constantly researching and reading everything I can on the subject. My nutrition education started long before I formally became a nutritionist.

I grew up in the 1970s, when meat, dairy, canned vegetables, and sugary cereals were considered essential for growing children. I never ate the meat, and I realized when I was very young that I didn't feel good after drinking milk. I noticed that when I wasn't feeling well I would crave fruit, and that after eating fresh fruit and vegetables, I would begin to feel healthy again. I began to read everything I could to find out about food (which, back then, meant going to a library).

This led me to years of experimenting with every food philosophy you could imagine. I feel that every food phase I travelled through taught me something important. When I tried going on a completely raw diet, I learned that a high fat raw food diet with a lot of nuts is difficult to digest and can often leave you feeling tired. I then went on to eating a lot of cooked vegan foods, mostly Indian, with coconut oil and coconut milk. This was followed by a spicy Mediterranean phase filled with tahini and hummus—not to mention all the dark chocolate along the way. As I was continuing my food journey, I always knew that there was a higher level of health to strive for.

Unfortunately, it seems that when we finally get to a point where we feel balanced in our body, life happens and we get stressed or sick and go back to what is familiar. Our old habits and ways of eating creep back in, and we end up consuming too much caffeine and sugary foods, making us once again imbalanced. I realized that achieving balance or homeostasis is an ongoing process and is not static. Think of yoga as an analogy: you are still moving when you are balancing in a posture.

My education in the field of food and nutrition and my years of experience seeing clients, writing, teaching and researching led to the book you now hold in your hands. My goal with this book is to take you on the same path I take my clients, towards better health, increased energy, and smoother skin. This book will not only help you reduce cellulite but will help you look and feel amazing, inside and out.

Different foods affect your body in different ways. It is important to focus on the actual foods you are choosing, especially the sodium and fat content and the combinations of the foods you are ingesting. Most importantly, you need to understand the effect different foods will have on your body.

Your body will always strive for health and no matter where you are presently it is never too late to make changes. As you get older, you come to realize the importance of hydration, sleep, food, healthy relationships, peace of mind, happiness and relaxation. Eating right for your body can be challenging, even for me, but once you understand the logic behind it, it makes it that much easier.

"To eat is a necessity, but to eat intelligently is an art."

The choices you make have a direct impact on the health of your body. What you eat, drink, breathe, think, and apply to your skin is how you bring the outside world in. When you stress, worry or think negative thoughts, your cells are listening as thoughts create neuropeptides—chemical signals—and every cell in your body has a neuropeptide receptor. This affects the functioning of your immune system and your overall health. Most of us chew and swallow our food without a thought of how it is going to be processed and utilized by our bodies. Digestion, absorption, and elimination are ongoing processes that we take for granted, as long as they go unhindered. When one of these processes becomes impaired, the body as a whole begins to suffer. Symptoms may not appear right away, but your body will give you clues including fatigue, bags under the eyes, obesity, excessive thinness, skin issues including cellulite and rashes, constipation, pain, stiffness, and headaches. You are constantly receiving messages from your higher self about your health, and by listening to these messages you can detect imbalances and help your body's ability to heal. When you refuse to listen to what your body is trying to tell you, your body will keep increasing the intensity of the message until you finally listen.

It is important to be aware of the substances you are putting into your body. Sometimes we discount what is best for us physically in favor of what feels right for us emotionally. We tend to justify and defend what we eat because of how we were brought up and our learned food habits. As a result, we habitually ingest foods that keep us in a limited version of ourselves. What we ingest is also one of the main contributors to the formation of that dreaded cellulite.

Eighty percent of women over the age of 40 suffer from the appearance of cellulite, so you are not alone. I will help you to understand the origins of cellulite and how you can diminish it. In order for that to happen, it will be important to make some lifestyle changes including eating a healthier diet, hydrating properly, exercising regularly, and following the other protocols I have outlined in this book.

This book is a result of my research, and yes, my personal experience with cellulite. Food is your medicine, but in order to truly heal your body, you also need a peaceful state of mind. If you follow my nutritional advice and add an exercise or yoga program, you will be thrilled with your results!

≈•≈ Ara Wiseman

How to Use this Book

This book was written to help you to understand the source of your cellulite and what you can do to diminish its appearance. As you read on, you will realize that cellulite is not a necessary part of your body. Cellulite occurs as a result of fat deposits being pushed through layers of weakened connective tissue under your skin. To treat cellulite successfully, you must make some lifestyle changes to reduce those fatty deposits, while strengthening the connective tissues in your body.

Once you begin to make these changes, you will start to see positive results. I wrote this book just for you, and in it I outline everything you need to know about making those changes.

Go through this book slowly, chapter-by-chapter, and let me help you understand how to diminish your cellulite. I provide plenty of options for you to make better choices to achieve positive results in your body—and ultimately in your life. Keep this book as a handy companion and refer back to it frequently for support and inspiration. Make your changes as you are able, knowing that you are actively taking steps towards creating a healthier, more beautiful you. What can be better than that!

- 1 -

The Importance of Hydration

Proper hydration is vital to the overall health of your body and its single largest organ, the skin. Two thirds of your body is comprised of water, which flushes out toxins, acts as an important catalyst in weight reduction, suppresses appetite, helps to clear waste, relieves constipation, helps maintain proper muscle tone, and helps to metabolize stored fat. Being slightly dehydrated can influence your mood and energy level and your ability to think clearly. Your digestive system uses several liters of water every day to process the food you eat. Consuming enough pure water will keep your skin soft and supple! If you didn't think drinking water was important, think again.

The liquids you drink should not be polluted with artificial sweeteners, sugar, caffeine or alcohol. It is best to drink filtered, purified water with some fresh lemon juice, greens powder or liquid chlorophyll.

HOW MUCH WATER SHOULD I DRINK EACH DAY?

It is very important to drink at least two to three liters of purified water every day to replenish the fluids your body loses through the normal activities of breathing, sweating, and elimination.

Drink 2–3 litres (8–12 glasses) of pure filtered water every day. Make it your goal to work up to that amount.

If you are overweight, physically active or live in a warm climate, you will require more water to help rebalance your body's fluids. If you have any symptoms of toxicity, you need to help flush out the toxins by making them more soluble. *Cellulite is a result of toxicity and poor circulation in the body.*

Your blood pressure and heart rate are affected by your level of hydration. A loss of just two pounds of fluid can increase your heart rate by eight beats per minute. This can affect your health and make you feel fatigued. Dehydration causes a drop in blood volume, forcing your heart to work even harder to move blood through your blood stream. Rhythmic movements of muscles like those that occur during yoga, will increase your blood flow, helping to lower blood pressure and improve circulation.

Dehydration can be responsible for headaches as a lack of water causes a vasoconstriction, a decrease in blood flow. If you suffer from headaches or migraines, try putting electrolytes such as Electro Mix or Emergen-C in your water. This can relieve most headaches, depending on their cause. These electrolytes come in little packets and can be found at most health food stores.

Often when people think they are hungry, they are actually dehydrated. Simply drinking enough pure water throughout the day ensures proper hydration, which can easily prevent that three o'clock head nodding at your desk. Sodas, coffee, and caffeinated teas will stimulate you for a short period of time but will let you down soon after. Think twice before you reach for any other fluid besides water! Invest in a stainless steel water container that you can carry with you everywhere; it will become your best friend.

MORE BENEFITS OF GOOD HYDRATION

The body's cells and connective tissues also require adequate hydration. The connective tissue can become dry and brittle, losing elasticity, and becoming weakened. This results in cellulite and aging skin. To strengthen your cells and keep the connective tissue healthy, commit to keeping yourself hydrated. Youthful skin is smooth and plump with properly hydrated cells.

Chlorophyll, helps to energize your body and eliminate toxins. It can also neutralize body odors and acts as a natural deodorant. Chlorophyll is non-toxic, soothing to the body's tissues and safe for use by people of all ages. Just add a few drops of liquid chlorophyll to your water!

Proper hydration is of utmost importance because water is the solvent that our body uses to transport nutrients and wastes. Without it the liver can't metabolize fat into usable energy, our connective tissue becomes weakened, we become constipated, and there is a build up of toxins. Our body then protects itself from excess toxins by storing them in our fat tissues. All this leads to that dreaded cellulite.

- 2 -

Free Radical Damage: How It Contributes to Cellulite

"It's really not time that ages you, but rather a lack of true nourishment on all levels." ~ Stephen Lau

So you have some free radical damage. The good news is that your body is forgiving and renewable. The best help you can give your body is to ensure your cells receive all the nutrients essential to cellular health, including antioxidants.

WHAT ARE FREE RADICALS?

To explain the term "free radical" requires a little bit of basic biochemistry. A free radical is an atom or group of atoms that has at least one unpaired electron, making it unstable and highly reactive. Free radicals can damage cells and accelerate the progression of cancer, cardiovascular disease, and many age-related diseases. Cellular damage is cumulative over the years, giving us the illusion that we age because of time. Free radicals actually speed up the process of aging by breaking down collagen.

WHERE DO FREE RADICALS COME FROM?

Free radicals come from many different sources.

From within ▎ They come from within the body as natural by-products of ongoing biochemical reactions. They occur during our normal metabolic functions and in the body's natural detoxification process and immune system defense.

From without ▎ Today, our toxic environment contributes enormously to the dissemination of free radicals. We are constantly being exposed to pesticides, insecticides, herbicides, air pollutants, UV rays, food additives, plastics, drugs, household cleaners, solvents, fire proofing agents, airplanes, radiation, fried foods, alcohol, tobacco smoke and so on, putting a toxic chemical burden of stress on our bodies.

Other sources of free radicals and factors that age our skin
Processed food and junk foods are high in sugar, sodium, and unhealthy fats. Unhealthy fats come from vegetable oils that are polyunsaturated and should not be heated, but in our Standard American Diet (SAD) usually are. Vegetable oils are high in omega-6 fatty acids and accumulate in the body, leading to inflammation and weight gain. They affect the thyroid and cause symptoms of hypothyroidism.

Sugar is highly acidic and gets stored as fat. It suppresses the immune system, decreases serotonin (your feel good neurotransmitter), is highly addictive and feeds cancer cells and yeast. The list of negative effects goes on and on.

Excess sodium in our diet can disrupt the required balance of potassium and sodium in our body. Numerous studies have demonstrated that a low potassium (K), high sodium (Na) diet plays a major role in the development of cancer and cardiovascular disease.[1] Today, most people have a potassium-to-sodium (K:Na) ratio of less than 1:2, which means they're ingesting twice as much sodium as potassium. To maintain optimum health, the ratio should be at least 5:1 potassium to sodium. Fruits and vegetables have a K:Na ratio of at least 50:1. Some examples are: apples 90:1, bananas 440:1, carrots 75:1 and oranges 260:1. When you consume too much sodium it can cause edema (swelling) in your body. It's important to aim for more potassium in your diet than sodium.

Burnt foods, especially barbecued meats, should be avoided. High temperature cooking, specifically burning the meat, creates chemical compounds called "heterocyclic amines" (HCAs), which are cancer causing.

Animal products, especially red meat, are acidic and produce inflammation in the body. The "heme iron" from meat gets absorbed, whether your body requires it or not, regardless of how much iron is already in your body—this is your iron status. Alternatively, the "non-heme iron" from plant foods utilizes a more selective absorption. If your body needs more, it will absorb more; if it needs less, it will absorb less. "Non-heme iron" has a built in regulatory mechanism based on your iron status and the other foods present in your diet. A high absorption rate is not a good thing because the body has no mechanism to dispose of the excess iron. "Heme iron" is absorbed in an unregulated way and accumulates over time in the body. This excess iron promotes free radicals and causes oxidative damage to the lining of the arteries, which may be a risk factor for cardiovascular disease, insulin resistance, and diabetes. Hormones are injected into livestock to increase milk production and lean body mass. Every time you eat commercially raised meat including beef, veal, poultry, pork, and lamb, you are consuming these hormones, which are harmful to you and your children in many ways. Roy Hertz, former Director of Endocrinology at the National Cancer Institute and a leading authority on hormonal cancers, warned specifically of the carcinogenic risks of estrogenic additives, which can cause imbalances and increases in our normal hormone levels. These hormones have an especially negative impact on growing children, who frequently end up entering puberty early as a result. Milk from commercially raised cows contains recombinant Bovine Growth Hormone, which has high levels of a natural growth factor known as IGF-1 (Insulin-like Growth Factor 1). This substance can survive digestion, remain in your body, is readily absorbed from your small intestine into your blood, and has been shown to cause cancer.[1]

Preservatives and chemicals are found in processed foods. One example is monosodium glutamate (MSG), which is considered an excitotoxin, and can be disguised in foods with its many nicknames. You may see it listed on a package as: MSG, hydrolyzed vegetable protein, hydrolyzed protein, hydrolyzed plant protein, plant protein extract, sodium caseinate, calcium caseinate, yeast extract, textured protein, autolyzed yeast, or hydrolyzed oat flour.

It is important to completely avoid consuming foods that contain excitotoxins, as they are chemicals that wreak havoc in your brain. You have a barrier protecting your brain but these chemicals are able to cross this blood-brain barrier, causing the brain cells to fire uncontrollably, eventually leading to cell death. Excitotoxins include any products containing aspartame, MSG and soy protein isolates, which are soy extracts found in a lot of vegetarian processed foods. Soybeans naturally contain high glutamate levels but when they are hydrolyzed, they release the free glutamate. Excitotoxins are dangerous for your body and have been implicated in dementia and brain atrophy.

Further effects of free radicals
In addition to all the aforementioned nasty effects of free radicals, they also wreak havoc on your skin (from both inside and out) resulting in diminished elasticity, uneven skin tone, age spots, and wrinkles. Two significant contributors to skin aging are the free radicals that come from cigarettes and over exposure to the sun's rays. Free radicals cause oxidative stress and damage the circulatory system, resulting in health related issues. Free radicals are also the main contributors of damage to your circulatory system which results in cellulite and other health related issues. To balance out these unruly molecules the body creates antioxidants whose sole purpose is to neutralize free radicals.

The good news is that within our cells we have protective mechanisms that nature designed to disable free radicals. They come with names like superoxide dismutase and glutathione peroxidase. In order to do their job, these enzymes require nutrients like manganese, selenium, and copper, which are present in whole grains, fruits, and vegetables. The bad news is that our body is only designed to create a certain amount of these antioxidants on its own. Today we are assaulted with an ever-growing number of environmental toxins, far more than the system designed by nature is able to handle. Overloaded with toxins producing free radicals, the body is simply not capable of handling all these harmful invaders, and we have to take action in order to help it out.

Glutathione is the major antioxidant produced by our cells. It works directly in the neutralization of free radicals and reactive oxygen compounds and maintains antioxidants such as vitamins C and E in their active forms.

Glutathione plays a role in the detoxification of many xenobiotics (foreign compounds) in our bodies. It is an essential component of the human immune response and can slow down the aging process.

As we age, glutathione levels decline. It is unclear whether this is because we use it more rapidly or produce less of it.

WHAT CAN I DO TO HELP MY BODY?

The first thing to do is to choose foods that are sources of glutathione. Fresh fruits and vegetables provide excellent levels of glutathione, but cooked foods contain far less or none at all. Asparagus is an excellent source; broccoli, avocado and spinach also boost glutathione levels. Undenatured whey protein is one of the best precursors (building blocks) for glutathione. Unfortunately, if foods that contain whey are heated or processed, they become denatured. Denaturation means that the natural structure of the protein has taken on a new structure, even if it is only slightly different. Heat and pH changes will alter the structure of the whey protein, and once this happens, the protein becomes denatured and will no longer help to build glutathione.

Immunocal (HMS 90) protein powder is a great source of undenatured whey protein, as it contains the building blocks needed for the production of glutathione in your cells. You can buy glutathione in capsule, pill or powder form, but if it does not contain the precursors, it will not be very effective. These precursors are the three amino acids: cysteine, glutamic acid, and glycine. Undenatured whey protein provides these three amino acids as well as many other amino acids and nutrients. You can find cysteine in alfalfa sprouts, red peppers, garlic, onions, broccoli, cabbage, brussels sprouts, oats, legumes, whole grains, sesame seeds, and mushrooms. Make sure to add a fiber source, such as ground flaxseeds, if using whey protein powders.

Other important antioxidants

The antioxidants naturally occurring in the plants—fruits and vegetables—we eat work in the body the same way they do in the plants. Plants produce the antioxidants, and when we eat them, we borrow their antioxidant shields and use them to support our own good health.

Antioxidants include vitamins A, C, E, Beta Carotene, Coenzyme Q10, Selenium, and Zinc. These nutrients are essential for your skin because they can slow the aging process by protecting collagen, the foundation for blood vessels and all connective tissues.

It's important to understand that antioxidants are most beneficial in whole food form because whole foods contain an assortment of nutrients that work synergistically together. Therefore, simply taking supplements is not the answer. The answer is to consume an abundance of organically grown fruits and vegetables. Organic green tea is also a good source of antioxidants although it contains caffeine, so make sure to consume water when drinking caffeinated beverages. To prepare green tea and preserve the antioxidants make sure the water is anywhere from 122°F – 175°F depending on the grade of the tea.

WHAT ARE PHYTOCHEMICALS?

Phytochemicals, also called phytonutrients, are health-protecting compounds found in fruits, vegetables, and other plants. They include beta-carotene, lycopene, resveratrol and anthocyanins, among others. The most powerful antioxidant known today is called astaxanthin. A member of the carotenoid family, it is derived from red algae and produced in Israel. Astaxanthin is the most powerful free radical scavenger as it is sixty-five times more powerful than vitamin C. It enhances our immune system, is anti-inflammatory, and discourages skin wrinkling. Research has shown that it can protect against DNA damage because it protects the entire cell. Food sources of carotenoids include: parsley, carrots, spinach, kale, winter squash, apricots, cantaloupe, and sweet potatoes.

Anthocyanins are a very large group of red-blue plant pigments that protect collagen. Members of this group include eggplant, acai, berries, cherries, and red grapes. These foods bolster cellular antioxidant defenses and help in the fight against free radical damage created by the sun.

Food sources of antioxidants

Vitamin A — Fruits rich in vitamin A include: apricot, cantaloupe, mango, orange, apple, watermelon, plum, blackberry, peach, and kiwi. Vegetables rich in vitamin A include: carrots, pumpkin, broccoli, peas, spinach, sweet potato, turnip, tomatoes, wheat germ, escarole, collards, dandelion greens, mustard greens, and aloe vera.

Vitamin C — Foods rich in vitamin C include: parsley, broccoli, bell pepper, cauliflower, kale, mustard greens, brussels sprouts, strawberries, oranges, papaya, and lemon juice.

Vitamin E — Foods rich in vitamin E include: mustard greens, chard, spinach, turnip greens, sunflower seeds, and almonds.

Selenium — Foods rich in selenium include: wheat germ, brazil nuts, oats, bran, red Swiss chard, barley, turnips, garlic, brown rice, crimini mushrooms, asparagus, sunflower seeds, and blackstrap molasses.

Zinc — Foods rich in zinc include: ginger root, rye, oats, buckwheat, almonds, pecans, walnuts, hazelnuts, Brazil nuts, sesame seeds, pumpkin seeds, lima beans, split peas, green peas, turnips, parsley, potatoes, and spinach.

It is important to always try to eat organically grown foods. If you choose conventionally grown produce, wash the fruits and vegetables with food grade hydrogen peroxide to remove any residual pesticides and herbicides. (*See the Dirty Dozen and Clean 15 Chart, page 170, for the list of the fruits and vegetables that are the most and least contaminated by pesticides*).

Free radicals wreak havoc on our body, especially our skin. As we age we become more susceptible to the effects of oxidative stress. Food that is anti-inflammatory and rich in antioxidants can slow the effects of aging at the cellular level. Reducing stress, obtaining adequate rest, practicing yoga and deep breathing, exercising, and making healthy lifestyle choices all slow down the aging process.

Adding lots of fresh fruits, vegetables, and greens such as wheatgrass, barley grass, alfalfa, kale, parsley, watercress, spinach, and collard greens is the best choice you can make for your body. These nutrient-rich foods are high in chlorophyll and give your body the energy it needs. The trick is to eat plenty of fruits and vegetables that contain an array of colors.

– 3 –

Collagen, Elastin and Strong Connective Tissues

WHAT ARE COLLAGEN AND ELASTIN?

Collagen and elastin are proteins contained within your skin that provide its structural integrity. Collagen is a fibrous protein found throughout your body, which gives your skin its firmness. Elastin is another type of protein, which keeps your skin flexible. As the name implies, elastin is elastic and works in partnership with collagen. While your collagen is busy providing firmness and rigidity, it is elastin that allows your connective tissue to stretch and then return to its original position.

The bad news is that as you age your body produces much less of these two valuable proteins, resulting in sagging skin and wrinkles. To compound this issue, free radicals, which are abundantly present throughout our environment, further the damage. In addition, as you age, the synthesis of glycosaminoglycans (GAGs) decreases, affecting the moisture levels in your skin. The result is that your collagen becomes brittle and dry and prone to breakage. It's important to make sure you are getting the foundational substances upon which your body's proteins are built. This will increase your skin's defenses against cellulite.

WHAT CAN I EAT TO INCREASE MY COLLAGEN AND ELASTIN?

The good news is that there are many foods that can help. It is important to eat fresh, organically grown foods that contain all the essential nutrients your skin needs for good health. Yes, it is all about fruits and vegetables.

Vitamin C ❏ According to The Linus Pauling Institute, vitamin C aids in the formation of collagen in your body to keep your bones, skin, tendons and tissues strong. Vitamin C protects the structure of your skin by repelling free radicals that damage collagen and elastin. To increase your vitamin C intake your diet should include fruits such as oranges, strawberries, and grapefruit, as well as vegetables such as broccoli, peas, sweet potatoes, and red bell peppers. Broccoli and brussels sprouts also contain a compound called Indole-3-carbinol (I3C), which helps to breakdown estrogen. Excess estrogen causes a multitude of symptoms and is one of the causes of cellulite. Researchers at the Linus Pauling Institute at Oregon State University found that the compound sulforaphane, which is found in cruciferous vegetables such as broccoli, bok choy and brussels sprouts, has strong anti-cancer properties. Broccoli sprouts have more than fifty times the amount of sulforaphane than mature broccoli.

If you decide to take a vitamin C supplement, the most absorbable form is liposomal vitamin C, which is bound to phospholipids. Liposomes are a matrix of microscopic fat particles made from phospholipids and has vitamin C contained within it. Since it closely resembles our cells, it easily passes through our intestine and into our blood, basically sliding directly into our cells. If choosing a liposomal vitamin C, choose one that uses sunflower seed lecithin instead of soy lecithin; there are a multitude of problems that arise from using soy.

Zinc ❏ Zinc is an essential mineral found in almost every cell and is necessary for the linings of the body, elastin and wound healing. Good dietary sources of zinc include: pumpkin seeds, ginger root, buckwheat, pecans, Brazil nuts, almonds, walnuts, hazelnuts, lima beans, split peas, and green peas.

Lutein ❏ Antioxidants like lutein can neutralize free radicals, preventing damage to your skin. Lutein helps to increase elastin (flexibility) in the skin. We get Lutein from green leafy vegetables (kale, spinach, collard greens, turnip greens), peas, broccoli, green beans, cucumber, arugula, and red grapes.

Vitamin A/Beta-carotene ❏ To maintain healthy and glowing skin you need to eat foods rich in vitamin A—*every single day*. Vitamin A is an antioxidant and one of the fat-soluble vitamins that can boost the production of collagen levels in the skin. There are two forms: retinol and beta-carotene. A healthy liver converts beta-carotene to vitamin A. However, people with diabetes and hypothyroidism (underactive thyroid) cannot convert beta-carotene to vitamin A, and therefore need to consume a direct form of vitamin A. Sources of vitamin A include: carrots, broccoli, sweet potatoes, chili peppers, dandelion root, collard greens, kale, parsley, spinach, mustard greens, dried apricots, mangoes, and cantaloupe. You can also apply a 1% or higher retinol vitamin A serum every evening on your face.

Copper ❏ Copper is an essential trace mineral and it is necessary for proper development of connective tissue and skin pigment. It is the third most abundant trace mineral, after iron and zinc. Copper is necessary for the proper function of the enzyme lysyl oxidase, which is required in the cross-linking of collagen and elastin.[2] Copper deficiency, therefore, is associated with poor collagen integrity.

Sources of copper include: Brazil nuts, almonds, hazelnuts, walnuts, pecans, split peas, and buckwheat. Avoid toxic forms of coppers that can be absorbed from meat contamination, second hand smoke, copper kettles and pipes, and acidic foods cooked in copper pots.

Vitamin E ❑ Vitamin E is a very effective antioxidant and is used by the lipid (fatty) portion of your cell membranes to stabilize and protect the integrity of those cells from the effects of free radicals. Good sources are nuts, seeds, whole grains, nut butters, and green leafy vegetables. The best form of vitamin E is alpha-tocopherol, which is found in the aforementioned foods and higher quality supplements. Synthetic vitamin E has only half the potency of the natural alpha-tocopherol.

Sulfur ❑ Sulfur is one of the most abundant minerals in the body and is found in your skin, hair, nails, connective tissue and nerve cells. As a component of collagen, it helps to keep skin cells supple and elastic. It also helps in the digestion of fats and controls the metabolism of carbohydrates. It is believed that sulfur helps to get rid of waste and poisonous matter from the system. Broccoli, cauliflower, kale, cabbage, and other cruciferous vegetables are rich in sulfur-containing nutrients called glucosinolates. Other sources include legumes, onions, garlic, shallots, leeks, and egg yolks. Sulfur is a component of amino acids and is present in most protein-rich foods.

Protein ❑ Protein gets broken down into amino acids, which are the foundational substances needed for the production of elastin and collagen and can assist in strengthening your skin's defenses against cellulite. The type of protein you ingest will have an affect on the condition of your skin. Proteins from animal sources are converted into uric acid and urea, which the body must then neutralize to prevent organ damage. The neutralized acids are impurities that end up on our hips, buttocks and thighs as cellulite.[3] The healthiest protein sources come from green leafy veggies such as kale, collards, spinach, bok choy, turnip greens, and beet greens.

Other sources of protein are legumes such as lentils, mung beans, adzuki beans, chickpeas, and kidney beans. If you are going to sprout legumes the best ones are lentils, peas (garden, sugar snap), and mung beans. Legumes contain anti-nutrients (substances that block the absorption of nutrients) such as hemagglutinins and trypsin inhibitors. Generally, the level of trypsin inhibitors in germinated legumes decreases the longer the legumes are sprouted and the seed then slowly releases its store of nutrients. The best sprouts are mung bean, alfalfa, sunflower, broccoli, and clover sprouts. Other preferred sources of protein are tempeh (fermented soybeans), sprouted organic tofu (in very limited amounts), mushrooms, asparagus, cauliflower, broccoli, millet, quinoa, buckwheat, brown rice, raw almond butter, raw nuts and seeds (especially pumpkin and sunflower seeds), wheat grass, barley grass, broccoli, and gluten free breads made with quinoa or buckwheat flour.

We don't require as much protein as we once thought. In fact, getting only ten percent of your calories from protein is sufficient. Excess protein puts a lot of stress on your kidneys and liver. Consuming a lot of protein increases insulin-like growth factor 1 (IGF1), which accelerates the growth rate of normal tissue and increases the growth rate of diseased tissues like cancer.

The Goji berry ❑ Goji berries contain antioxidants that improve circulation and are a great source of protein. They contain eight amino acids and twenty-one trace minerals. According to Dr. Murad in his book *The Cellulite Solution*, "Goji berries are nature's cellulite assassins."[4] They contain high amounts of vitamin C and are rich in essential fatty acids. You can buy them dried, eat them alone, add them to trail mix, or put them on top of salads.

Essential fatty acids ❑ EFAs are "essential" because the body doesn't manufacture them. We need to consume foods that contain them or take them in supplement form. EFAs are anti-inflammatory and attract water for our connective tissues. Fatty acids seal the moisture barrier in every cell to protect them from water loss and dryness. You will find high amounts of essential fatty acids in hempseeds, hemp oil, flaxseeds and flax oil. *Both these polyunsaturated oils should be consumed raw—never heated.* EFAs are also found in walnuts, chia seeds, and green leafy vegetables.

Milk thistle and dandelion ❑ Milk thistle seeds contain an antioxidant bioflavonoid complex known as silymarin. They can be ground into cereals or smoothies. Milk thistle may protect the cells of the liver by blocking harmful toxins and helping to remove them. Your liver is responsible for executing over five hundred functions and will always benefit from a gentle cleanse. The results of a liver cleanse may include increased energy, fat and weight loss, reduced cellulite, clear skin, reduced Premenstrual Syndrome (PMS) symptoms, and many other benefits. Dandelion is another herb that is nourishing for the liver and is also a diuretic. Its main mineral is potassium, which helps to reduce water retention. You can also add a few dandelion greens to your salad or you can drink it as a tea.

Ginger ❑ Ginger is anti-inflammatory and aids in circulation, which is helpful in cellulite reduction.

An Ayurvedic Tea to Combat Cellulite:
    1/4 tsp raw fresh ginger
    1/4 tsp dill seed
    1/4 tsp fenugreek seed
    1 clove
    Cover with 8 oz. boiling water for five minutes.

HOW CAN YOU PREVENT CELLULITE FROM FORMING?

Spend less time sun tanning ▮ A certain amount of sunlight is healthy, but lying in the sun for hours is not. Excess sun exposure, also known as photoaging, can break down and damage collagen and elastin in your skin, causing premature skin aging, wrinkles, uneven skin tone, dark spots and rough, dry skin.

Certain medications, like birth control pills and hormone therapy, may increase the skin's photosensitivity to direct sunlight and can result in pigmentation problems.

Keep yourself hydrated ▮ It is important to drink plenty of water. Try adding a greens powder, fresh lemon, or wheatgrass. Harsh weather, dry air, wind, and extreme heat or cold can deplete your skin of essential moisture, resulting in dry lines. Adequate hydration is the antidote. Sea Buckthorn oil, applied every day under your moisturizer, is amazing for your skin. It contains an omega-7 fatty acid that will help reduce wrinkles and dry skin. It can also be taken internally for weight loss as it signals the body to stop storing fat.

Stop smoking ▮ Smoking depletes the body of vitamin C and can prematurely break down collagen, resulting in sagging skin and wrinkles. Tobacco smoke is loaded with toxins that increase free radical damage, which then has to be neutralized using up precious mineral reserves. Smoking also significantly decreases the supply of oxygen to your skin cells.

Avoid/reduce stress ▮ Stress, anger, and worry will create wrinkles and over time can lead to health issues. Stress depletes our adrenal glands of much needed adrenalin, leading directly to exhaustion and eventual illness. Stress negatively affects our metabolism, blood sugar balance, and immune system. When we experience stress, we are in our "fight or flight" response and start functioning from our sympathetic nervous system. When we eat in this state, we cannot digest our food properly. Proper digestion occurs when we are relaxed, and functioning from our parasympathetic nervous system. Stress and anger deplete the body of vitamins B and C and interfere with digestion.

Are you worrying yourself to wrinkles? Your brain doesn't know if something is real or perceived, so if you are worrying or thinking negatively then your brain will register it as a real threat and send a cascade of hormones throughout your body in response to it. This changes your internal biochemistry. Over time, elevated stress levels deplete you of nutrients, creating an imbalance and leaving you feeling depleted.

Get enough quality sleep ▌ Lack of sleep adds to stress, irritability, depression and fluctuations in growth hormones.[5] Evidence links lack of sleep to obesity, increased inflammation and lowered immune system function. While you sleep, your skin is being renewed and restored. If you have a bad night of sleep, the effects are immediately noticeable in the appearance of your skin. Researchers at Cornell University found that stress and lack of sleep had an impact on the skin's barrier function, which increased water loss from the skin and is one of the causes of cellulite.[6]

Avoid consuming alcohol ▌ Excessive alcohol consumption causes dehydration in the body's cells, which can accelerate premature aging. Alcohol depletes your body of vitamins B and C along with essential fatty acids. Alcohol metabolism produces toxic by-products, leading to more free radicals, affecting the structure and appearance of the skin. These toxic by-products need to be eliminated from the body as quickly as possible. Too much consumption causes damage to the liver and depletes the adrenal glands. Alcohol can suppress the appetite, causing fewer nutrients to be consumed and absorbed, once again affecting your skin.

Avoid consuming sugar ▌ Sugar is a highly addictive substance. Sugar depletes the body of minerals, impairs hormonal function, and depletes serotonin (our feel good neurotransmitter). It is highly acidic because once it is consumed, sugar converts into acetic acid. Sugar attaches to the collagen protein in our skin and forms Advanced Glycation End Products (AGEs). The acronym AGE is fitting, since it ages us from the inside out. This causes cross linkages, "molecular handcuffs," either inside or outside your cells, impairing the cells structure and altering its ability to function, ultimately leading to damage. Once glycated, collagen has a reduced regenerative ability and shows up on your skin as wrinkles, sagginess, decreased elasticity, and discoloration or brown spots. These cross linkages are what cause the stiffness and inflexibility in your body.

Avoid consuming caffeine ▌ You love your morning coffee or your favorite breakfast tea, and who doesn't love chocolate? But watch your caffeine consumption—caffeine is addictive, and that's just the beginning. The caffeine found in coffee, tea, cola, chocolate, and some medications can not only lead to addiction, but also to adrenal depletion, hypoglycemia, and vitamin B deficiency. Caffeine actually dehydrates your skin which promotes aging. Coffee and black teas have been shown to reduce the absorption of iron and zinc. A few hours after drinking a coffee, once the blood sugar has dropped, most people reach for something sweet. This causes daily fluctuations in energy levels and over-stimulates the adrenals, leading to fatigue, adrenal exhaustion, weight gain and a decreased ability to handle stress. Cut down on caffeinated drinks and choose healthier options like herbal teas, fresh juice, or purified water.

Exfoliate ❙ Exfoliating your skin with exfoliating creams or by dry brushing will eliminate dead skin cells from the surface layer of your skin. Dry skin brushing helps with lymphatic drainage, and exfoliating actually stimulates the production of new elastin and collagen.

Deep breathing ❙ Start to become mindful of your breathing. Stress can cause a multitude of symptoms and leads to shallow breathing, using only twenty percent of your lung capacity. Shallow breathing then leads to poor circulation and more tension. Breathing deeply can help you relax. Your breath purifies your blood, provides you with more energy, calms your mind and body, and transports life-giving oxygen to all parts of your body. Your body must have oxygen to cleanse itself of waste, making oxygen one of the most important nutrients. While the brain needs the largest amount, every organ and cell in the body requires oxygen to function, including your skin, which is rejuvenated by oxygen. When the body doesn't receive enough oxygen, there is a lack energy and vitality.

The science of breathing is called "pranayama." "Prana" is a Sanskrit word meaning the ever-present life force. "Ayama" means to extend and release. Pranayama breathing is traditionally done early in the morning, but can be practiced at anytime, depending on your lifestyle. Choose a quiet place to practice deep breathing exercises daily.

The value of deep breathing is priceless. The breath carries oxygen in and removes metabolic waste via the lungs. For this to happen, the breath must be deep enough and slow enough. Most people breathe with very little attention to the length and efficiency of their breath.

A simple yet powerful breathing exercise can supercharge your breathing pattern in the short term, or it can become a wonderful habit, reaping benefits for decades to come.

A Deep Breathing Exercise and Meditation

- Sit comfortably on a chair with both feet on the floor or sit cross-legged on the floor or use a meditation pillow. The coveted lotus position (with both knees on the floor) is beyond the reach of most people, and not necessary for short sittings. Supporting your back by sitting against a wall or the back of a chair may be helpful in the beginning.
- Imagine a point of light residing in the bottom of your spine, at the tailbone. As you inhale through the nose, bring that light up gently all the way to the top of your head. Then as you exhale through the mouth, with your lips gently opened, bring the point of light back down to the tailbone. Do this slowly, gently, focusing on the light's pathway, the spine. As you inhale, you will start feeling very light and even a bit warm. Enjoy it. As you exhale you will feel rested and grounded.
- Do not hold your breath; just switch from inhale to exhale as soon as you feel the lightness, then switch back to inhale as soon as you need to take the next breath.
- Do six to twelve cycles of this breathing exercise. Then, rest for two to three minutes without paying attention to your breath at all. Open your eyes or continue towards meditation, if that is your practice.
- Meditation is a wonderful tool to keep your mind cool and calm. Once you learn how to do it and begin to practice meditation regularly, it will help you even during the craziest storms in your life.

- 4 -

How Much Body Fat Should I Have?

The objective for weight loss is to lose fat, not muscle. Research has shown that a person with an apple-shaped body (more weight around the waist) is prone to more health risks than someone with a pear-shaped body (more weight around the hips). Either way, carrying extra weight is not healthy. Fat produces estrogen, causes inflammation and stores toxins. A certain amount of body fat is needed to cushion the vital organs and insulate them from the cold, ensuring that the body does not shut down important functions in order to maintain proper body temperature.

Body fat assists with the utilization of fat-soluble vitamins. Women typically carry six to eleven percent more body fat than men. Studies have shown that estrogen reduces a woman's ability to burn energy after eating, resulting in more fat being stored in her body. The likely reason for this is to provide support for the menstrual cycle, childbearing, breastfeeding, and changes in hormone levels. Fat storage points are partly genetic and partly hormonal. Our hormones are responsible for where fat gets deposited; around the pelvis, buttocks, and thighs for women, and around the belly for men.

The ideal percentages for body fat are 12 – 20% for men, and 18–28% for women. However, the following factors determine how much body fat loss is attainable and optimal for your body, and why fat loss can be slow and stubborn to lose.

Age ... Metabolism begins to slow down after age twenty-five, mainly due to lifestyle factors. During midlife, hormones affect the rate of calorie burning, so it is important to be realistic about weight loss goals.

Medication ... Some medications slow down the metabolism, further slowing down fat loss.

Body composition ... Muscle is more metabolically active than fat, therefore, increasing your lean body mass will increase your metabolism.

Hormones ... Insulin, thyroid, adrenal, estrogen, and growth hormones all play significant roles in fat and calorie burning.

Gender ... Men burn 30% more calories than women, both at rest and during exercise.

Nutritional status ... A low calorie, nutrient-deficient diet decreases the metabolic rate by 10 – 20% or about 150 – 300 calories daily. Nutrient deficiencies affect calorie burning by not having the needed enzymes and co-enzymes available for assimilation, repair and elimination. Yeast or fungus in your body affects metabolism, as they feed off of the nutrients and reduce the chemical and mechanical absorption of everything you eat by at least half.[7]

HOW TO INCREASE YOUR METABOLISM

Exercise ▌ Your metabolism is affected by the amount of body fat vs. lean body mass you have. Did you know that your muscle burns fat even at rest? One pound of muscle actually burns an additional fifty to one hundred calories per day, so it's important to increase your muscle mass. You can do this with resistance training (using rubber bands, a stability ball or light weights), pilates, and yoga. Find an exercise program or yoga routine that you enjoy and can stick with. Walk as often as possible and take the stairs instead of the elevator whenever possible.

Get adequate sleep ▮ The hormones that regulate our appetite are influenced by the amount of sleep we get. Ghrelin and leptin are two of the hormones that affect hunger, and their levels tend to vary at different times. Leptin, a hormone released by our fat cells that controls our appetite and signals satiety to our brain, is dependent on our sleep. Chronic sleep deprivation can create a shortage of leptin, altering its effectiveness and making us feel hungrier. Ghrelin is a hormone produced by the stomach that sends us a signal when we're hungry. When we are awake, more ghrelin is produced. Lack of sleep affects these hormones and their ability to accurately signal our caloric needs. That is why people often put weight on when they are sleep deprived.

Balance your hormones ▮ Stress causes an imbalance in our hormones. When you are experiencing stress, your cortisol level goes up. Elevated levels of cortisol, estrogen and insulin turn on galanin, a neurotransmitter that makes you crave the unhealthy fats in foods such as ice cream, chocolate, potato chips, and hamburgers. Another neurotransmitter, neuropeptide Y (NPY), is triggered by stress. As NPY levels go up, so do the cravings for sweets.[8] Improving your nutrition and making lifestyle changes that move you towards reducing or managing your stress levels and detoxifying your body will help restore your hormonal balance.

Increase potassium ▮ Start to focus on eating more fruits and vegetables to increase the amount of potassium in your body. This will help to correct any tissue damage that has been caused by excess sodium. According to Dr. Max Gerson, when there is a loss of potassium our cells will try to maintain their integrity by binding sodium with water. This causes fluid retention or edema that damages our cells. Healthy cells have a high ratio of potassium to sodium whereas diseased cells have an abundance of sodium or a low ratio of potassium to sodium.[9]

Here are three ways to increase your potassium and energy levels:

1. Drink pure water with a greens powder or liquid chlorophyll added.
2. Make sure 3/4 of your plate is filled with dark leafy greens and vegetables (steamed, raw, sautéed or baked).
3. Use your juicer. Juicing dark leafy greens like kale, collards and spinach and using parsley, coriander, sprouts, cucumbers and celery is an excellent way to increase nutrients and energy. (*See Healthy Juices, pages 134–135*).

Regulate your blood sugar levels ▌ Your liver, pancreas and adrenal glands regulate your blood sugar. These organs and glands become taxed by chronic stress and the consumption of sugar, refined carbohydrates, caffeine, and alcohol, resulting in blood sugar imbalances. Blood sugar regulation equals willpower. If your blood sugar is continuously fluctuating, it is difficult to avoid caving in to sugary temptations. Incorporating more fiber rich foods, whole grains (gluten free preferably), ground flaxseeds, legumes and vegetables will help to stabilize your blood sugar levels. Reducing your fat consumption is also necessary to stabilize your blood sugar.

Strengthen digestion ▌ Your colon represents 70% of your immune system, so keeping it clean is of the utmost importance. Poor digestion contributes to creating a toxic colon, which will affect your skin. Your colon needs at least 25 grams of fiber every day, and enough water to form and remove stool.

Take a good probiotic ❙ Taking probiotics, the good bacteria, is a great way to keep the bad bacteria in check. Some good sources are Udo's Choice, Genestra HMF or Metagenics, which you can find in the refrigerator section of your health food store. These good bacteria produce lactase for lactose breakdown and help to metabolize cholesterol to prevent re-absorption, thereby lowering it. They manufacture B vitamins and vitamin K and inhibit toxic nitrates (found in luncheon meats) from becoming cancer-causing nitrosamines. In addition, they enhance bowel function while decreasing acne and other skin problems. It's important to select a good probiotic, and take it every day.

Reduce your anxiety ❙ Our cells listen to our thoughts. When we worry or think those 'what if' thoughts, they register in the limbic system, also known as our emotional nervous system. The limbic system is integral to all the activities essential to our self-preservation and it records our stresses along with all the feelings and sensations in our body. The hypothalamus translates the messages from the limbic system and then sends a message to the immune system and the pituitary, which regulate our hormonal system. This causes changes to the hormonal balance in our body, causing our entire endocrine system to change. An imbalance in our adrenal hormones will create a greater susceptibility to disease. Therefore, it's essential to be mindful of what we're thinking about, since our cells listen to our thoughts.

THINGS YOU CAN DO TO IMPROVE YOUR DIGESTION

Chew your food well ❙ If you chew your food until it is a paste, it will lessen the amount of work required by the rest of the digestive system. Chewing also helps you relax. Digestion is linked to relaxation via the parasympathetic nervous system, so if you eat while you are anxious or stressed, you will not digest your food properly.

Learn to eat slowly ▌ Eating slowly allows your digestive system to communicate satiety to the brain. Over-eating slows down your digestion, resulting in a sluggish digestive system, lethargy and weight gain.

Enzymes ▌ We are what we digest and assimilate. Avoid eating foods that you are sensitive to. Most people find taking a plant-based digestive enzyme with heavier meals to be helpful. Bitters, such as gentian root or Swedish bitters, will stimulate your digestive juices including saliva, stomach acid, and bile. Bitter greens such as dandelion, endive, and radicchio are also helpful for digestion. Cold beverages with meals numb the stomach's acid producing glands, which in turn will inhibit digestion for several hours. Instead, drink plenty of pure, room temperature water in between meals and throughout the day. After meals, avoid drinking caffeine. It stimulates the emptying of the stomach before your food is completely digested. This may prevent the absorption of important nutrients.

Practice proper food combining ▌ Simplifying your meals makes them easier for your body to digest. The fewer types of foods you combine, the better your digestion will be. The salivary juices in the mouth digest carbohydrates, while the acidic juices in the stomach digest proteins. Eating a heavy meal of protein (especially meat) and starches (rice, bread, potato, and pasta) takes longer to digest. Separating your starchy carbohydrates from your proteins will improve your digestion, free up energy and speed up your metabolism. Animal protein must be broken down (hydrolyzed) into simple amino acids before the body can use them. This process robs the body of vital energy and that is why most people are tired after eating a steak. Plant proteins are simple structures of amino acids, which require less energy.

The sweeter or more refined the carbohydrate (white bread, cookies, cake, pie, chocolate) the more it interferes with stomach acid. When you eat fruit, you need to consume it on its own, on an empty stomach. Eating protein with sweets, including fruit, directly after a meal should be avoided. Sugars are digested in the intestine but proteins and fats remain in the stomach for hours. If you eat fruit after eating other food, it will mix in your stomach with the protein and fat, and can cause gas, bloating, and fermentation. A lot of raw foods are made predominately from fat (nuts, nut cheeses, flax crackers), which lingers in your bloodstream for many hours. Excess fat will inhibit proper digestion, creating elevated blood sugar levels.

Eat the right food for your body ▌ Eat healthy, satisfying meals so you can avoid late night snacking. Don't under eat fruit, including sweet fruit, in general; they are so healthy and full of nutrients. You need to allow your body to finish digesting the previous meal before eating the next one. The key is to choose healthy foods, and avoid foods that you are sensitive or intolerant to. Bloating, gas, discomfort, sluggishness, headaches, inflammation, and irritated skin are just a few symptoms of food intolerances.

Fasting ▌ It is important to give your digestive system a break. Since fasting is difficult for most people, start by not eating after dinner. In the morning have a couple glasses of water and fruit for breakfast, and a fresh vegetable juice or more fruit for lunch. This is a great way to give your body a chance to eliminate and focus on internal housecleaning. If you start by doing this once a week, you can begin to decipher what your body really needs.

Eat foods like apples ▌ Apples contain an insoluble and soluble fiber called pectin, which is found in the cell walls of fruits. Pectin absorbs watery substances, which bombard the cells, forcing them to release fat deposits. An apple a day keeps the fat at bay.

Eat foods high in vitamin C ▍ Oranges, tangerines, grapefruits, lemons, and limes contain a high concentration of vitamin C. Vitamin C reduces fat by liquefying or diluting it, thereby making it easier to flush out of your system. Vitamin C is an essential cofactor for L-carnitine, a metabolism boosting amino acid. One function of L-carnitine is to shuttle fat molecules to the site of fat oxidation in tissue cells, where they are broken down to release energy. When carnitine concentrations are reduced, fat tends to accumulate in tissues.

Incorporate ground flaxseed ▍ Flax seed contains five grams of soluble fiber per tablespoon and is the ideal source of alpha linolenic (ALA), the fatty acid essential for efficient metabolism. ALA also helps to protect the cells' integrity and is anti-inflammatory. Aim for at least three tablespoons of ground flaxseeds each day.

Incorporate chia seeds ▍ Chia seeds are high in fiber, omega-3 fatty acids, calcium, antioxidants, and protein. Chia contains 11 grams of fiber per ounce and absorbs up to 12 times its own weight. You can put two tablespoons of chia in one liter of filtered water overnight in the refrigerator. In the morning squeeze in some fresh lemon juice and enjoy. It is not only healthy but will curb your appetite and help you start to focus on eating more fruit and less refined carbohydrates. Chia seeds have more omega-3 fatty acids than salmon and without heavy metals. Essential fatty acids (EFAs) are the basic building blocks of every cell in our body and an integral part of our cell membranes. Our body needs fatty acids to rebuild and create new cells and regulate various processes in our body. Our body cannot manufacture them; they must be supplied through our diet. They also support heart health and beautiful skin.

Always eat to nourish yourself ❙ We are what we eat because after we assimilate the food, it becomes a part of us. Our food should be organic, close to the way nature made it, unprocessed, non Genetically Modified (GMOs) and preservative free.

Avoid dairy products ❙ Dairy products are full of hormones, contaminants, and unhealthy fat and cause an immune system response. Dairy is highly acidic, and most people are lactose intolerant and cannot properly digest dairy. From my experience with clients, dairy can exacerbate acne and cellulite.

Remove or lessen obstacles that interfere with healing and cellulite reduction ❙ Avoid white sugar, alcohol, caffeine, tobacco, recreational and pharmaceutical drugs. Try to limit exposure to harmful air pollution, electromagnetic radiation from cell phones and computers, especially WiFi.

Many factors are detrimental to our wellbeing, including overeating, overworking, stress, lack of exercise, sunshine, and fresh air. Repressed emotions such as regret, guilt, sadness and self-destructive attitudes and thought patterns are harmful. These are all indications and reminders that we need to slow down, be in the moment, and learn to see the challenges we face as opportunities for growth. We can then find healthy solutions to overcome them by welcoming the experiences we are currently going through, knowing they are there to teach us something about ourselves. Be grateful for everything, as there are hidden blessings in every struggle we face.

– 5 –

How to Reduce Excess Fat

Perhaps you have been hiding those tenacious folds on your belly, cursing the rolls on your legs and the wings you have somehow developed underneath your arms. Some of us might only have a few inches to lose or some dimples to get rid of, but some of us need a bit more of a concentrated effort to fit into our favorite dresses and jeans. What should we do?

You will need a daily plan that is comfortable, sustainable, delicious, and nutritious. The food you eat should be nutritious and tasty, simple to prepare, and easily attainable anywhere.

WHY POPULAR DIET APPROACHES ARE HARMFUL AND DON'T WORK

You might have tried a low fat, low carbohydrate, high protein diet. In the short run those diets can produce weight loss, however, in the long run, this is the most dangerous diet. Protein is not a clean fuel for energy, and when you consume too much of it, your organs will suffer greatly from it. High protein diets have been shown to increase the body's stress response by increasing cortisol levels and lowering our calming neurotransmitter GABA, that is associated with well-being, proper memory function, circadian rhythms, and sleep by quieting your brain. *High protein diets can cause anxiety, stress and mood disorders.* Too much protein in your diet will keep your blood saturated with acid byproducts that result from its breakdown.

This overworks the buffering systems in your body, which can lead to negative health consequences. Our buffering systems are at work all the time neutralizing the acids that are formed from our normal metabolic activities. Therefore, it is best to avoid a highly acidic diet that creates unnecessary work, and can overtax your system. Our body will store excess acids in our fat cells, so even if you are losing weight your dreaded cellulite is still there. It is not uncommon to see slim women with dimples on their legs, the back of their arms, and even on their belly. Men have cellulite too; it shows up as bumps and globs of fat just under the skin.

A low fat, high carbohydrate diet can be difficult for some people to maintain because of the low fat recommendations, especially if you don't have the right information or an understanding of the science. Our taste buds get accustomed to the high fat and sodium in foods, which sets us up for cravings. With the proper low fat, high carbohydrate foods, maintenance is easy, keeping you healthy and feeling energized with smooth, clear skin. Many of us have been misled to believe that whole fruits are the culprits in weight gain, which is a common fallacy. Fruits are full of vitamins, minerals, antioxidants and fiber, and have the highest electrical energy of all foods. The more you consume energetic foods, the more vibrant and healthy you become. Fruits are astringent and help to tighten our tissues. Sour citrus fruits such as lemons and limes, cleanse our tissues and increase the absorption of minerals. According to Dr. Robert Morse, fruits are brain and nerve foods that help to clean our tissues. Vegetables are considered the builders and are great for muscle and skeletal tissue, while raw nuts and seeds (fats) are structural foods that strengthen the whole body. It is important that you consume raw, ripe fruits and lots of fresh vegetables in order to regenerate your body, including your skin.

WHAT *SHOULD* I BE EATING?

The answer is fresh fruits, vegetables, sprouts, whole unprocessed grains (preferably wheat free), legumes, and a limited amount of nuts and seeds. Yes, you read it correctly, lots of fresh fruits and vegetables with limited healthy fat will keep you slim and cellulite free, safely and beautifully, for the long run.

Whether you want to keep your body in perfect health or you have a chronic condition, including heart disease, arthritis, diabetes, or chronic fatigue syndrome, it is imperative to keep both your fat and your protein intake to 10 percent each of your total calories. That means reducing your consumption of oils and switching to vegan, plant based protein sources. The healthiest vegan protein sources are green leafy veggies, such as kale, collards, spinach, bok choy, turnip greens, and beet greens. Other sources include organic tofu (in limited quantities), tempeh, raw nuts and seeds, and legumes such as lentils and beans, which will require a little more energy to break down. When your protein and fat intake are each 10 percent of your daily calories, carbohydrates will make up the remaining 80 percent.

Healthy carbohydrates come from whole foods such as fruits*, vegetables, unprocessed gluten free grains, and legumes. The best carbohydrates for reducing cellulite are fruits and vegetables. The best gluten free grains are quinoa, buckwheat, and millet. Try to avoid eating too much bread, even if it is gluten free. Root vegetables, including squash, sweet potato, and potatoes are healthy complex carbohydrates that contain valuable fiber and protein with minimal fats.

---

*Fruits are best eaten away from complex carbohydrates and fats, but they do combine very well with green leafy vegetables.

Fat makes our food tasty and keeps us satiated for hours, but not all fat is created equal.

Most saturated fat is from animal origin, and you want to stay away from it. Just like humans, animals store toxins in their fatty tissues. Once you know this, you can choose to avoid animal fat.

In addition to animal fat, you need to stay clear of trans fat. Any polyunsaturated fat that is heated will become a trans fat. Most processed food and store bought vegetable oils contain rancid fat. Most restaurants will fry the food repeatedly in the same oil, creating toxic trans fat. Trans fat increases your chances of developing degenerative diseases and interferes with the metabolism of the good essential fat that you need. They are absolutely everywhere and ingesting them is one of the biggest problems in today's diet.

Most people consume far too much fat, and according to Dr. Neal Barnard, M.D., "Everything changes when you eat fatty foods, or when you gain a significant amount of weight. Insulin can't work in an oil slick. When there is too much fat in the bloodstream, insulin's hand slips on the knob. Unable to open the door to the cells, sugar builds up in the blood. Your body responds by making more and more insulin and eventually it will get the sugar into the cells." This causes blood sugar disorders. The problem is that most people will blame the fruit. It's not the fruit that is to blame, but the overall diet that is too high in fat and most likely too high in protein. Fructose is found naturally in fruit and does not require insulin or extensive digestive enzymes. It is easily metabolized, giving you more energy, whereas a lot of food tends to take energy from us. Do not mistake naturally occurring fructose from fruit with high corn fructose syrup (HCFS). HCFS is a highly processed unnatural sweetener made from corn and is highly toxic. According to Dr. Morse, N.D., "Fructose from fruit does not require insulin to be carried through a cell wall, it is merely pulled in by diffusion."

What about oil?
Oil should not be considered a health food. Whole foods are stripped of their fiber, protein and carbohydrates when they are processed into oils, leaving an imbalanced food that is 100% fat. Concentrated oils are high in calories (approximately 120 calories per tablespoon) and low in nutrients.

The best way to consume fat is in small amounts naturally found in whole foods. Raw nuts and seeds and their butters, avocados, olives, and young coconut flesh with all their nutrients still intact are excellent sources of healthy fats. The fiber in whole plant foods helps to keep fats from going rancid and creating oxidative damage to our cells, one of the key causes of cellulite and skin-aging.

What is a beneficial essential fat?
The best fat contains essential fatty acids (EFAs) and comes from plant sources. Some of the best-known sources are flax, chia, hemp seeds and walnuts. Surprising to most people, green leafy vegetables are an excellent source of EFAs. If you are using hempseed or flaxseed oil, make sure that these oils are cold pressed and stored in dark containers to protect them from heat, light and air. Buy the smallest container available and store it in the refrigerator to avoid rancidity. Omega-3 and omega-6 oils belong to a very special class of poly-unsaturated fats. Flax and hemp oils are rich in omega-3s, which are chains of carbon with available places where molecules can bind, thus helping to lubricate our cells, joints, brain and other vital organs. For healthy and happy cellulite-free living, include very small amounts of these oils daily. Some good brands are Barlean's Organic oils and Manitoba Harvest. These oils are sold in an optimal ratio of omega-3 and -6 fatty acids and should be taken daily as a supplement, rather than a condiment. Again, they must never be heated.

These essential fatty acids play an integral role in the health of our skin. We must get them from our food, as we cannot synthesize them within our body. A small daily dose of healthy fat is a sure way to build up your immunity, protect your brain from aging, reduce inflammation and help your skin stay youthful and soft. Who doesn't love silky smooth skin?

What are the healthiest and safest fats to heat?
When it comes to high heat cooking low sodium vegetable stock is the best choice and will help you to eliminate the need for oil. If you are using oil, then coconut oil is your best choice. Over 90% of the fatty acids in it are saturated, which makes it very resistant to heat. This oil is semi-solid at room temperature and it can last for months without going rancid. Coconut oil is rich in a fatty acid called lauric acid, which helps kill bacteria and other pathogens. You can use it as a moisturizer on your skin or hair; it keeps your skin healthy and youthful looking.

Unrefined virgin olive oil is a monounsaturated fat but contains 14 – 17 percent saturated fat. It is best not to heat this oil. Using this oil in its purest form is the most beneficial. Extra virgin olive oil is best consumed raw, in salads or added to cooked foods once they have cooled off. Remember though, it is best to keep your fat intake to 10 percent of your calories and that may mean eliminating oils.

The best sources of monounsaturated fats come from whole food plant sources such as avocados, almonds and other nuts and seeds. Almonds, walnuts, cashews, and all the other nuts are easier to digest when they are made into butter using a stone grinder or a blender. Soaking almonds overnight will neutralize or minimize the enzyme inhibitors and make them easier to digest.

Grape seed oil is rich in omega-6 fatty acids, and is 70 percent polyunsaturated. It must be cold-pressed organic grape seed oil (not chemically pressed), so that it retains its nutrient profile. Non-organic grape seed oil contains pesticides and other chemicals. Unfortunately, the refined and chemically processed grape seed oil that is readily available contains toxins left behind during processing.

Grapeseed oil is less volatile at higher heat levels than other polyunsaturated oils, so you can cook with it, but not at high temperatures.

It is important to keep oils/fats away from the complex carbohydrates because there is a long process to break down the complex carbohydrates and the oils will slow this process down even further.

How to take care of edible oils

In order to make sure that your fats and oils don't go rancid, it is important to keep a few things in mind. Don't buy large batches at a time—buy smaller ones, that way you will most likely use them before they get the chance to go rancid. The main causes of oxidative damage of edible oils are heat, oxygen and light. Keep unsaturated fats like olive, hemp, and flaxseed oils in the refrigerator and make sure to screw the lid on as soon as you're finished using them. There are flax and hemp oils that come with lids that you can squeeze the oil through, without having to remove them.

Why cold-pressed?

Although slightly more expensive, it is best to choose oils that are cold-pressed. They are subjected to less heat than commercial, solvent-extracted oils and lower heat means less breakdown of nutrients. They are processed without the use of solvents, eliminating any potential for toxic residue.

GREEN LEAFY VEGETABLES ARE THE REAL SECRET

Another major element to achieve cellulite-free living is plenty of green leafy vegetables. That deep green color is the secret to a very healthy diet, along with healthy fruits, colorful vegetables, and pure water.

Kale, collard greens, dandelion leaves, spinach, romaine lettuce, and the many varieties of green leafy lettuce, including Boston, butter, escarole, and mache are excellent blood builders and support a healthy immune system. These wonderful plants contain plenty of protein. Eat them raw in salads, juice them, steam them lightly, blend them into a soup or add them as a topping to already cooked soups.

Colorful vegetables that are botanically classified as non-sweet fruits, like peppers, tomatoes and cucumbers are also a very important addition to a healthy diet. Cucumbers are electron rich, have a high water content and are considered both a fruit and a vegetable. They make the perfect base for green smoothies or vegetable juices. All these vegetables are acid buffering and very nutrient dense foods. They deliver plenty of the vitamins and minerals we need daily.

OTHER WONDERFUL FOODS

Let me introduce you to a wonderful food that is available all year around. It is tasty, very nutritious, low in sugar and calories and costs only pennies per pound. Have you guessed it yet? Sprouts! Yes, these tiny little shoots are very powerful. When we eat them raw and unprocessed, they deliver vitamins, minerals, and other essential nutrients to our cells. They make any salad majestic and any sandwich light to bite into. Many grocery and health food stores carry sprouts, but due to their very fragile nature they can spoil easily. Before you buy, you should examine them carefully to ensure the little buds are green or white, not brown and yellow.

But the best way to get your sprouts is to grow them yourself in jars or trays. All you need is water and light. Rinse and spray three times a day, and in three to five days a whole pound of fresh green sprouts greet you. Once they finish growing, they can be stored in the fridge for up to five days.

Broccoli, bok choy, cabbage and other vegetables rich in sulfur will give your diet a boost. Steam them, shred them raw onto a salad or put them into a green shake.

> **Sample Day of Meals**
>
> *Breakfast*
> Green shake or fresh fruit until lunch—fruit must be eaten on its own, on an empty stomach.
> (*See Green Shakes page 136.*)
>
> *Mid morning*
> Green shake or fresh fruit, or celery and carrot sticks with some homemade low fat pesto, hummus or guacamole.
>
> *Lunch*
> Raw or cooked soup, gluten free flatbread with grilled vegetables and sprouts on top.
>
> *Mid afternoon*
> Green juice, barley grass with coconut water or shake.

Dinner
Salad with colorful veggies, a few vinegar free olives, homemade dressing made from fruit, or raw tahini and lemon (*Chapter 18, Recipes*), steamed veggies with a little tamari. Add a lentil burger or any of the vegetable burgers on pages *153, 158, 159.*

Healthy Dessert (*pages 164 – 165*).

How Toxicity Contributes to Excess Body Fat

Our modern lifestyle and eating habits create toxins and impurities in our bodies. Fortunately, we have buffering systems working all the time that neutralize acids and keep our blood and fluids in the normal range. There is a lot of talk about the alkalizing and acidifying effects of different foods. Foods leave either an acid ash or an alkaline ash once they are metabolized. Your body keeps your blood pH between 7.35 to 7.45 and the foods that you are eating are not causing any large deviations in your blood pH. Eating an unhealthy diet of processed foods, fast foods, animal products, soft drinks or alcohol, which are mainly acid forming, can stress and overwork your buffering systems, affecting your energy levels, skin and overall health.

When there is an overabundance of toxins and impurities, the body tries to neutralize them by using up its own mineral reserves. For instance, one of our buffering systems requires calcium phosphate salts which are found in the structural components of our bones and teeth. Calcium is one of the most abundant minerals in the body and buffers the onslaught of acids, protecting our organs, tissues and cells. Over time this leads to mineral deficiencies.

These neutralized acids are eliminated through your colon, kidneys and skin, but when there is an excessive amount, not all of them can be eliminated at once. Your body will then store these toxins in your fatty tissues. For women, these fatty deposits put pressure on the connective tissue and weaken it. These underlying fatty deposits push through the weakened connective tissue and create cellulite. Excess fat produces inflammation, causing a cascade of problems. Acids and toxins consume our mineral reserves, leading to mineral deficiencies.

From my experience, when mineral deficiencies exist we tend to feel a void. We then crave and eat more of the wrong foods trying to fill it. In North America this can be considered "affluent malnutrition," because even though we have an abundance of food, millions of people are malnourished, literally starving for vitamins and minerals. This starvation is a result of people consuming too much protein, animal fats, coffee, cigarettes, alcohol, soft drinks, sugars, pastries, and processed foods loaded with additives and preservatives. All this makes the problem worse and perpetuates the cravings and addictions. It deteriorates our health and beauty and seriously impacts our emotional state and behavior.

Acid production occurs through normal body processes such as digestion, respiration, metabolism and cellular breakdown. We must help the body by consuming alkaline foods rather than adding to the problem by consuming acidic foods and drinks.

Here is a list of the acids produced in your body after eating some very common foods.[10]

Meat and meat products	Uric acid
Pork	Sulphuric and nitric acid
Sweets, sugar, white flour products	Acetic acid
Artificial sweeteners	Formic acid
Soft drinks	Phosphoric acid
Coffee, black tea and red wine	Tannic acid
Pain relievers	Acetylsalicylic acid
Physical overexertion	Lactic acid
Stress and anger	Hydrochloric acid

FOODS AND WHAT THEY LEAVE BEHIND

Here's a little chemistry lesson:

✐ Acid-ash foods leave high concentrations of chloride, phosphorus and sulfur. The body uses these minerals to make acids like hydrochloric acid, phosphoric acid and sulfuric acid.

✐ Alkaline-ash foods, on the other hand, leave high concentrations of magnesium, calcium and potassium. These minerals are used to form alkaline compounds called bases, including magnesium hydroxide, calcium hydroxide and potassium hydroxide.

WHAT ARE ALKALINE FOODS?

A foods acidity and alkalinity is based upon its mineral content. It just so happens that fruits and vegetables, which are alkaline, are also the healthiest foods. Consuming more foods that are alkaline is healthier for your body. Below is a chart of foods to help you. After reading the list, you might wonder how you are going to give up some of your favorite foods. Remember that your body's buffering systems are continuously at work keeping your blood pH tightly regulated, so the food you are eating is not affecting the pH of your blood but can affect your energy level and the look of your skin. In order to not overwork your buffering systems it is important to focus on choosing healthier options. It is just a matter of becoming aware of and changing your daily habits. Start by cutting down on oil/fat, calories, the majority of your carbohydrates can come in the form of fruit and vegetables. There are recipes and a meal plan at the back of this book to help get you started. Just so you know, every 35 days your skin replaces itself and your body makes new cells from the food you are eating. The food becomes a part of you as you metabolize, assimilate, and absorb the energy it provides into your own energy. Food enters into you, dissolves within you, penetrates your cells, contributes its energy to you, and therefore becomes you—it is the most intimate of connections. We must feed ourselves with love, and be mindful of what we consume.

If you are reasonably healthy, your diet should consist of 70–80% alkaline-forming foods and 20 – 30% acid-forming foods to maintain your good health. If you are unwell in any way, your diet should consist of 80% alkaline-forming foods and only 20% acid-

ALKALINE FOODS		ACIDIC FOODS	
Vegetables Asparagus Artichokes Cabbage Lettuce Onion Cauliflower Radish Green leaf lettuce Peas Red cabbage Leeks Watercress Spinach Turnip Chives Carrot Green beans Beetroot Garlic Celery Grasses (wheat, barley, alfalfa, kamut etc.) Cucumber Broccoli Kale Brussels sprouts Squashes Earth/root Vegetables	**Fruits** Lemon Lime Avocado Tomato Grapefruit Watermelon (is neutral) Rhubarb **Drinks** Green drinks—greens powder; chlorella, spirulina, grasses; wheat, alfalfa, kamut, liquid chlorophyll pH Drops for water or Alca base powder with alkalizing minerals, cell food. Fresh vegetable juices Pure water (distilled or ionized) Lemon water (pure water + fresh lemon or lime). Herbal teas	**Meats** Pork Lamb Beef Chicken Turkey Crustaceans Other seafood **Others** Vinegar White pasta White bread Whole wheat bread Biscuits Soy sauce Tamari Condiments (tomato sauce, mayonnaise etc.) Artificial sweeteners Honey	**Dairy Products** Milk Eggs Cheese Cream Yogurt Ice cream **Drinks** Fizzy drinks Coffee Tea Beer Spirits Fruit juice Dairy smoothies Milk Traditional tea

forming foods, to help restore your health. You can accomplish this by increasing your intake of fruits and vegetables, vegetable juices or by using green powders.

ALKALINE FOODS

Sea & Root Veggies & Mushrooms	Drinks
Kombu	Homemade vegetable broth
Nori	Non-sweetened homemade almond milk
Wakame	**Seeds, Nuts & Grains**
Daikon	Almonds (can be soaked in pure water overnight)
Dandelion root	Pumpkin
Squash	Sunflower
Maitake	Sesame
Chaga	Flax
Reishi	Buckwheat groats
Cordyceps	Spelt
Shitake	Lentils
	Cumin seeds
Umeboshi	Any sprouted seed; all sprouts are extremely healthy
	Millet
Fats & Oils	**Others**
Flax and ground flaxseed	Sprouts (soy, alfalfa, mung bean, wheat, little radish, chickpea, broccoli etc)
Hemp and ground hempseed	Bragg Liquid Aminos (Soy sauce alternative)
Avocado	Hummus
Olive oil	Tahini
Evening primrose	
Borage	Fermented tempeh
Coconut oil	
DHA from algae	All seaweeds

ACIDIC FOODS

Convenience Foods	Fats & Oils
Sweets	Saturated fats
	Hydrogenated oils
Milk Chocolate	Margarine (worse than butter)
Microwave meals	Corn Oil
	Vegetable oil
Canned foods	Sunflower oil—Stay away from all vegetable oils except the ones listed under Fats & Oils under Alkaline foods.
Powdered soups	
Instant meals	
Fast food	
Fruits	**Seeds & Nuts**
Fruit is extremely healthy and full of nutrients and antioxidants. Fruit must be eaten alone on an empty stomach. Fruits digest quickly, but when combined with other foods, their sugars are held up in the stomach, resulting in fermentation.	Peanuts
	Cashew nuts
	Pistachio nuts

ALKALINE FOODS

General Guidance:

Make sure to eat plenty of fresh raw vegetables and healthy nuts and seeds. Only use the oils listed, especially coconut oil because it contains healthy properties and is the safest oil to cook with. Make sure to drink plenty of pure water daily with a greens powder, wheat grass, or chlorophyll.

Fruit is also an essential part of a healthy diet, so make sure to include a lot of fresh fruit, preferably ripe and in season.

ACIDIC FOODS

General Guidance:

Steer clear of fatty meats, dairy and cheese, sweets, milk chocolate, alcohol and tobacco. Packaged foods are often full of hidden offenders and microwave meals are full of sugar, sodium, preservatives and chemical additives. Not to mention that microwaving denatures your food. Over cooking also removes all of the nutrition from a meal.

Cleansing by cleaning up your diet can help remove the debris that has accumulated in your body over the years from environmental toxins, chemicals, excess refined food, fat, sugar, salt, colas, caffeine, alcohol, tobacco, animal protein, dairy, pharmaceutical drugs, artificial sweeteners and preservatives. Over time, these toxins harm your body causing low energy, pain, constipation, cellulite and inflammation, all of which lead to more serious health conditions.

The most highly acidic foods are all the animal foods—meat, eggs, dairy and cheese. After they are digested, they leave an acid ash that the body is forced to deal with. This leads to calcium loss and deficiency. Soft drinks have a pH between 2.8 and 3.5 and are a complete waste of energy. These liquid calories provide absolutely no nutritional value and cause a lot of damage to your body. Sugar is highly acidic and leads to acid build-up in your body, affecting the health of your bones as it eats away at them. And, just so you know, wheat is the most damaging of all grains.

In addition to all the dietary changes you can make, drink plenty of pure water, avoid excessive stress, get plenty of exercise and focus on the positive! Every new day is an opportunity to change and get healthier. I read somewhere that you will never change your life until you change something you do daily. The secret of your success is found in your daily routine.

HOW DO I KNOW IF I'M EATING THE RIGHT BALANCE?

To achieve a 70% alkaline to 30% acid balance, you don't have to measure your food, just look at your plate.

Make sure most of your plate is a large delicious salad with lots of different vegetables and some fun healthy dressings (*Chapter 18, Recipes*). Experiment with different herbs, seasonings and greens. The other 30% can include vegetarian dishes (perhaps a vegetable stir-fry), buckwheat soba noodles, brown rice or lentil pasta, quinoa, legumes, stew, or soup. Stay away from fast food. You can also include healthy gluten free breads or gluten free crackers. A word of warning—many gluten free products are made with a lot of starch, white rice flour and other ingredients that are not the healthiest. Read the labels and don't eat too much bread in general. Avoid eating bread daily, as it's not the healthiest choice and only adds the inches. If you are looking for a healthy bread choice, I suggest Littlestream's Quinoa Bread—it's healthy and gluten free or bread made with a sourdough culture. Always choose breads made with wholesome ingredients.

It's important to drink water throughout the day. Use liquid chlorophyll, greens powder, fresh or frozen wheat grass and barley grass.

GREENS POWDERS AND GRASSES

Greens powders are highly concentrated nutrition, packed full of vitamins, minerals, protein, fiber and chlorophyll. I would highly recommend Athletic Greens for your daily greens powder. Freshly juiced organic greens are the preferable choice. If time and resources are a factor, a greens powder is beneficial and recommended daily.

Wheatgrass and barley grass are healthy choices for the same reasons all green vegetables are. Wheatgrass is chockfull of nutrients, including iron, vitamins B, C, E, K, and high levels of vitamin A.

Grasses help to balance blood sugar levels and add minerals. They contain chlorophyll, which helps to deliver oxygen throughout the body, thereby building healthy blood cells. The molecular structure of chlorophyll is similar to human hemoglobin, but chlorophyll has magnesium in its center as opposed to iron.

As your taste buds start to decipher the taste of real foods and your system becomes accustomed to this way of eating, you will lose your cravings for unhealthy foods. I know that at this point it seems daunting to change routines and habits, but believe me, within a very short period of time you will feel better and look great!

The healthier your body gets, the more energetic you will begin to feel, not to mention the fat loss and reduction in cellulite that will occur. When you indulge in sugar and foods that contain a lot of fat, you will quickly notice a downward shift in your energy level, making you feel tired and sick.

Also a more fruit and vegetable rich diet is packed with nutrients and considered "nutrient dense" as opposed to calorie dense. This diet is more satisfying for your body and reduces food cravings.

For cellulite therapy to be as effective as possible, it requires a multifaceted approach. Here are some strategies and activities necessary to remove toxins and reduce cellulite.

- Incorporate the above foods and grasses into your diet.

- Reduce both your fat and protein intake each to 10% of your calories. Once you reduce fat you can start to consume fresh sweet fruits in higher quantities.

- Eliminate acidic foods.

- Become aware of your food addictions, emotional eating habits, energy level, mood and overall health.

- Stay hydrated by drinking at least one to two liters of water with greens, to flush out waste products.

- Bathe regularly in alkaline minerals or Epsom salts.

- Sweat out toxins using Far Infrared sauna treatments.

- Rebound on a mini trampoline at least fifteen minutes per day.

- Exfoliate every morning before you shower.

- Increase circulation through regular exercise and daily yoga.

- Get adequate rest and sleep.

- Detoxify regularly to strengthen the metabolic functions.

- Reduce stress.

- Enjoy fresh air and sunlight.

- 7 -

Insulin and Body Fat Regulation

If you carry excess fat you may experience blood sugar imbalances. These may show up as dizziness, tiredness, excessive thirst, brain fog, and intense cravings for sweets (the wrong kind of sweets). On a high fat diet, your bloodstream contains excess fat that impedes the movement of sugar out of your bloodstream. Fats take longer to eliminate, lingering in the bloodstream for many hours. Fat cells are involved in manufacturing and storing estrogen, so carrying too much fat increases your estrogen levels, leading to hormonal disruptions all over the body. If the liver is overburdened from too many toxins it can't eliminate the excess estrogen properly, resulting in belly fat and cellulite.

> *Here's an interesting fact*
> Fat cells are greedy and elastic as they can hold 62% fat, while other cells contain only 20% fat. While a person of average weight has about twenty-five to thirty-five billion fat cells, an obese person may have one hundred to one hundred and fifty billion! When we gain weight, fat cells puff up like little balloons until their capacity is reached. In order to store the extra fat more

fat cells are produced. Once fat cells are made, they are yours for life; they can grow or shrink, but they are now a part of you. Women carry body fat in their breasts, hips, buttocks, thighs, and waist. Men carry fat in their chests and abdomen.

THE HORMONE CORTISOL

Abdominal fat cells grow in response to insulin and cortisol. Cortisol is a stress hormone produced by the adrenal glands and is released in higher quantities when the body is reacting to stress. When there is chronic stress, cortisol signals the fat to be deposited in the abdominal region.

High cortisol levels cause blood sugar problems, sleep issues, reduced bone density, excess fat accumulation, high triglyceride levels, chronic fatigue, and suppressed immunity. High cortisol levels also shut down digestion and digestive secretions and shunt blood away from the gut. Nutrient turnover is increased while antioxidants, B vitamins and minerals get washed out of the urine.

Cortisol has a natural daily rhythm. Your body produces more in the morning, providing the energy you need to begin your day. Ideally, your cortisol level should drop by 90% in the evening, when you leave your stresses of the day behind.[11] Elevated cortisol levels at night will prevent or interrupt your sleep.

When your adrenals become exhausted from chronic stress, your thyroid will jump in to help and can become underactive (hypothyroidism). This leads to an imbalance in hormones resulting in low energy, weight gain, constipation and cravings for stimulants, including salt, sugar, junk food, coffee, or other caffeinated beverages. As you can see, our hormones work together like an orchestra.

To reduce fat

Increase mineral rich foods ❙ Eat lots of greens and drink plenty of water with wheat grass or one of the grasses for chlorophyll. Minerals will help with reducing cravings.

Avoid foods that stress your body ❙ Chief offenders include caffeine, artificial sweeteners, soft drinks, chocolate, junk foods, alcohol, white flour products, wheat (gluten), sugar, and fried foods.

Avoid consuming excess caffeine ❙ Its diuretic effect depletes B vitamins and overworks the adrenals. This in turn creates more physiological stress and exhausts the body's coping mechanisms.

Avoid sweets ❙ Insulin raises cortisol levels and high glycemic foods such as soft drinks, refined starches and sweets will elevate blood sugar and insulin levels, especially at night.

Increase your intake of fruits and vegetables ❙ They contain vital antioxidants, vitamins and minerals.

Consume essential fatty acids ❙ They are anti-inflammatory and important for your body and adrenal glands.

Take a magnesium supplement ❙ This will help relax you in the evening. Try Calm, a drink containing magnesium citrate or drink teas such as chamomile and passionflower to help calm your body.

Exercise ❙ Start to exercise because it will block the effects of cortisol by using the glucose circulating in the blood stream and it releases endorphins. Yoga is a great way to increase strength and calm your mind.

Manage your stress ▍ Stress raises cortisol levels. Stress is implicated in every symptom we experience and sets the stage for chronic illness.

Practice deep breathing techniques ▍ This will help with digestion, relaxation and keeping your mind calm and clear.

Get sufficient sleep ▍ Lack of sleep raises cortisol levels. Waking at two A.M. and not being able to get back to sleep can be caused by adrenal weakness, which is caused by stress.

Develop a positive body image ▍ How you feel about yourself can influence your body composition. When you have negative thoughts about yourself, your body releases cortisol, which mobilizes lean body mass, reduces the basal metabolic rate, redistributes fat, and ages the body.[12]

– 8 –

Healthy Blood Vessels

Healthy blood vessels are essential for proper circulation so that your blood is able to provide nutrients to all the different vital areas of the body. This is essential for collagen formation. The narrowing of the arteries due to plaque build up causes poor circulation. The nutrients in the blood become inefficiently transported, allowing only a small percentage to reach the body's cells. When this happens, your connective tissue will weaken and cellulite will appear.

To improve circulation, you *must* move your body to increase your heart rate by exercising, deep breathing, rebounding, doing yoga, being sexually active, or going on a vigorous walk. A bath in Epsom salts or dry brushing is also helpful.

- *Dry brushing*
  The skin is the largest organ in the body and dry brushing is one of the best techniques to open up the pores, stimulate circulation and detoxify the lymphatic system. It helps to increase blood supply to the surface of the skin, along with nutrients and oxygen. Dry brushing helps shed dead skin cells, which can help improve skin texture and cell renewal. When dry brushing daily, this technique can help prevent conditions like eczema and psoriasis from occurring and helps to diminish cellulite. When the pores are not clogged

with dead cells and the lymphatic system is clean, the body is able to eliminate toxins and waste materials in an efficient manner.

Purchase a natural bristle brush (not a synthetic one) with a long handle so it can reach all areas of your body. A brush with a removable head and a strap for your hand is ideal. Brush your dry body once a day, preferably in the morning, prior to your bath or shower. Begin brushing your skin in long sweeping strokes, starting from the bottom of your feet upwards. Move up from your hands towards your shoulders. Brush your torso in an upward direction, towards the heart. If you have cellulite on your buttocks and thighs, remove the brush from the handle and brush in circular motions. This will increase blood flow, bringing nutrients to the area.

DIETARY AND LIFESTYLE CHANGES THAT CAN CONTRIBUTE TO IMPROVED CIRCULATION AND HEALTHY ARTERIES

Things to avoid
1. Make sure to avoid rancid fats including supermarket oils that have been heated to high temperatures, rendering them rancid. Buy raw, unsalted nuts and seeds as they contain polyunsaturated fats that should not be heated (or roasted). Store them in the refrigerator to keep them fresh. (*Refer to Chapter 5 for good and bad oils.*)
2. Avoid trans fatty acids. They damage the endothelium (inner lining of the blood vessels), thus reducing the nitric oxide production in the vessels. Nitric oxide signals the smooth muscle to relax, resulting in dilation (expansion) of blood vessels to

increase blood flow. Reduced nitric oxide is the cause of blood vessel damage and consequently heart troubles.
3. Avoid all saturated fats, which means all animal products.
4. Avoid all the toxins listed in chapter three: *Cigarettes, pesticides, herbicides, household chemical cleaners, etc.*
5. Avoid rich, greasy foods, refined sugars, excess caffeine, white flour products, and chemical additives in food and water.
6. Eliminate the dietary abuses and habitual behaviors that destroy nutrients in the body: overeating, hurried eating without chewing properly, obsessive or mindless emotional eating, late night eating, or consuming fast food.

Things to include
1. Start eating whole healthy fats as opposed to oils, such as avocado, coconut, and raw nuts and seeds including flax and hemp.
2. Increase foods high in vitamin C and bioflavonoids in your daily diet. One of their main functions is to scavenge the free radical compounds, which damage cell membranes. Citrus fruits are high in vitamin C and act as a natural blood thinner. Hesperidin, rutin and narignin are the principal citrus bioflavonoids, which are found in fresh (not bottled or frozen) lemon, grapefruit, and orange juices, along with other bioflavonoids. Blueberries and raspberries provide bioflavonoids, which are natural compounds that help strengthen blood vessels. Bioflavonoids work with vitamin C and other nutrients in the body to help make capillaries less fragile. The darker the color of the fruit, like blackberries and cherries, the more bioflavonoids they have. The white membranes of citrus fruit, such as oranges and grapefruit, are also a rich source of bioflavonoids. They strengthen and protect collagen, the main protein in our connective tissue. Increasing vitamin C levels will also increase collagen formation.
3. Cayenne and turmeric improve blood circulation. Cayenne warms

the body and increases blood flow. Turmeric is anti-inflammatory and is a blood thinner. This bright yellow spice is a powerful medicine that has been used in Chinese and Ayurvedic medicine as an anti-inflammatory agent to treat a wide variety of conditions.

4. Ginger stimulates the blood flow to all organs and is anti-inflammatory.
5. Garlic is a natural blood thinner and improves circulation. Garlic also kills yeast or any fungus in your system.
6. Raw nuts and seeds contain healthy fats and are high in zinc and magnesium. Deficiencies in these minerals are linked to lowered immune function, anxiety and heart disease. Buy only raw nuts and seeds, and store them in the refrigerator to prevent them from going rancid.
7. Pumpkin seeds are anti-parasitic and high in zinc and vitamin E.
9. Celery helps to regulate blood pressure, as it dilates blood vessels. Celery is considered the "sexiest" vegetable. It contains vitamin E, magnesium, niacin, potassium, and zinc—all required for optimal sex. Celery also contains arginine, a natural amino acid that expands blood flow, much like Viagra. According to Andreas Moritz, a natural health expert, celery also contains two steroids: androsterone and androstenol. Research shows that the subtle odor of these two chemicals attracts the opposite sex. Just a few stalks every day can enhance your sex life!

A FEW WORDS ON SALT

Sodium is important for the body's proper water balance. It is needed for many bodily functions such as nerve and muscle function. There is a difference between sodium chloride (table salt) and sodium that occurs naturally and abundantly in whole plant foods. Eating a variety of vegetables especially celery and tomatoes, provides all the sodium, minerals, and nutrients our body requires.

Many people consume excessive levels of sodium, which causes edema, dehydration, high blood pressure, liver and kidney disease, or potassium deficiency. The body requires a delicate balance of sodium and potassium in order to maintain good health. When too much sodium is consumed, more potassium is needed for proper balance.

Potassium protects many body systems, including the kidneys, bones, and the cardiovascular system. Potassium is found in all fruits and vegetables, especially dark leafy greens. Foods high in potassium include, dark leafy greens, Swiss chard, spinach, romaine lettuce, asparagus, crimini mushrooms, lima beans, potatoes, brown rice, celery, squash, tomatoes, collard greens, avocado, broccoli, carrots, oranges, strawberries, apricots, bananas, papaya, and cantaloupe. While these foods are excellent sources of potassium, cooking them lowers their levels. Eating a raw salad and fresh fruits daily is the best way to keep your body in proper balance.

When we consume whole natural foods, we don't have to worry about getting too much sodium, fat, or sugar. The body is designed to derive optimal nourishment from whole, natural foods. The amount of fiber found in fresh fruits and vegetables is exactly the right amount for your body's needs. Incorporate a lot of fruit into your daily plan. The magnetic (electrical) energy found in fruit is the highest of all foods, making it a superior brain and nerve food. Fruit brings energy to the body, while many other foods take it away. Fruit has high amounts of antioxidants and enhance the vitality of our cells. Always eat fruit alone and on an empty stomach, do not eat fruit after a fatty or starchy meal. Fruit can be your best internal broom, sweeping you clean of old debris.

– 9 –

Maintaining Healthy Cell Membranes

Every cell in your body is surrounded by a cellular membrane, or wall, which is actually a semi-permeable filter through which nutrients can enter and wastes can be excreted. Cell membranes help to keep healthy nutrients in and pollutants out, and allow cells to communicate with each other in order to orchestrate all of the body's physiological functions.

The average adult has around thirty trillion cells. Every day thousands of new cells are made to replace the old cells as they die. These old worn-out or damaged cells are then added to the pile of internal toxins lining up to be eliminated. In order for your body to successfully remove these toxins, you need to be well hydrated. Providing your cells with all the required nutrients from the foods you ingest will help to rebuild them. In addition to our own metabolic wastes, in today's world we are continuously subjected to environmental toxins like herbicides, pesticides, insecticides, xenoestrogens from plastics, fast foods high in sodium and preservatives, excess sugar, air pollution, and stress. In a desperate attempt to protect itself from being over-loaded by all these toxins, your body stores them in your fatty tissues. These toxins will stay there, until you take action to mobilize and remove them.

The food you consume and ultimately assimilate has a major impact on the health of your cells.

Without the right nutrients, water and phytonutrients, your cell membranes can become weakened, develop holes, become leaky and not function properly. Over time, the cell walls can become even further damaged or more porous, allowing precious water to escape. In this damaged state, they are no longer able to attract or hold onto the water or the nutrients needed to function properly. The result is a loss of elasticity in the skin. The skin becomes dehydrated and wrinkled with visible cellulite.

WHAT NUTRIENTS DO WE NEED FOR OUR CELL MEMBRANES?

The cellular membrane is primarily composed of fatty acids held together in a phospholipid bilayer, which forms a barrier to keep the cells stable. Your cell membranes need good sources of essential fatty acids (EFAs), protein, a full range of vitamins, minerals including choline, phytonutrients, antioxidants, and water. All these wonderful building blocks are naturally available from the plant kingdom.

The role of essential fatty acids
Your cell membranes need healthy omega-3 essential fatty acids. "Essential" means that your body does not manufacture them, so they need to be obtained from food. A deficiency of essential fatty acids impairs cell membrane function. Since the basic function of the cell membrane is to serve as a selective barrier to regulate the passage of molecules in and out of the cell, a disturbance in this function will disrupt the cell's ability to control its internal environment.

Omega-3 essential fatty acid is alpha-linolenic acid (ALA). ALA is the foundation of the "omega-3" family of fatty acids. These essential fats are very volatile, meaning they are heat, light, and oxygen sensitive. It is absolutely imperative that these fats *never be heated*. Food sources of omega-3 include ground flax seeds, chia seeds, and green leafy vegetables.

In our modern world, we are bombarded every day with omega-6 fatty acids from vegetable oils, soy products, and from eating meat from animals that have been fed corn and soy. Too much omega-6 leads to inflammation and can affect your thyroid. This will affect your metabolism, which will, among other things, slow down your weight loss efforts.

When you eat unhealthy saturated fats, or trans-fatty acids, these fats also become part of your cell membranes. They are more rigid and wreak havoc on your body by slowing down the circulation of your blood. Once you have built up a fair number of fat cells, it is extremely difficult to get rid of them. These fat cells are very hungry, and each dietary mistake will feed them, thus allowing them to hang around.

The role of protein

Protein is a major component of your cells. It is located in the cell membrane, within the cell itself, and around the cells. Your cells are in constant communication with each other, taking in nutrients from your bloodstream and getting rid of wastes. Together with the good fats, protein maintains the integrity of your cell membranes, the pathways that can be opened and closed to transfer information when your cell gets the signal.

Healthy protein comes from plant sources, including green vegetables such as spinach, peas, broccoli, green beans, collard greens and kale. Plant foods deliver significantly more protein per calorie. Other good sources are apricots, prunes, guavas, dates, apples, avocados, green leafy vegetables, root vegetables, cauliflower, asparagus, mushrooms, legumes, quinoa, buckwheat, millet, raw nuts and seeds, wheat grass, barley grass, tempeh, and non-GMO sprouted tofu (in small amounts). For a more complete list, refer to the chart on pages 171–172, "Where Do I Find My Protein?".

As you can clearly see, it's imperative that your body gets the right nutrients in order to keep the cellular function running smoothly. Not getting enough essential amino acids (protein), essential fats, and nutrients results in unstable membranes incapable of keeping their buoyant shape. The health of your cell membranes determines how quickly your skin ages and the structural integrity of your tissues, which impacts, you guessed it, cellulite development.

The role of nutrients
Vitamin A ❏ Vitamin A and its co-factors will ensure smooth cell function. The best sources of vitamin A are green vegetables, root vegetables, tomatoes, carrots, turnip greens, broccoli, asparagus, avocados, pumpkin, watermelon, apples, apricots, prunes, papaya and lemon grass. Vitamin A is not affected by heat or light.

Vitamin B ❏ Vitamin B complex supports the nervous system and the adrenal glands, helping in overall stress management. Consuming whole grains, nuts and seeds, preferably in sprouted form (sunflower sprouts), will ensure a continuous supply of this essential water-soluble vitamin. As a water-soluble vitamin, it is easily flushed out during stress, strenuous exercise, alcohol consumption, and emotional upheavals.

Vitamin C ❏ Vitamin C is essential. Since it cannot be manufactured in the intestines, you must consume it in your foods. It is an antioxidant, thus helping the immune system. Your body needs vitamin C to make collagen, the "glue" that strengthens many things like your skin, muscles and blood vessels. Vitamin C gets rid of visible bruises easily, is great for wound healing and aids in bile production, which greatly enhances digestion of fats in the diet. The best sources are citrus foods such as organic oranges, mandarins, tangerines, clementines, and lemons. Other vitamin C sources include microgreens such as wheatgrass, barley grass, alfalfa, pea shoots and sunflower greens. Green leafy vegetables, romaine, arugula, kale, broccoli, collard, mustard and turnip greens, are excellent sources of vitamin C.

Choline ❏ Choline is a component of our cell membranes. Since cell membranes are almost entirely composed of fats, the membranes' flexibility and integrity depend on adequate supplies of choline rich foods. It is needed in the regeneration of our skin cells and protects our cells. It is a component of our nerve and brain cells and is helpful for memory. It is also helpful in reducing body fat and helps to move fat and cholesterol through the blood so it doesn't accumulate in arteries. Sunflower lecithin is the preferable choice over soy lecithin.

Vitamin E ❏ Antioxidants from vitamin E protect the cells from free radicals, boost the immune system and repair DNA. This vitamin is found in whole grains, some leafy greens like sunflower greens (sprouts), broccoli, asparagus, avocados and peas, as well as raw nuts and seeds and their raw oils.

– 10 –

The Hormone Connection

Youthful skin is smooth and plump with properly hydrated cells. It has a lot to do with a bountiful supply of the fluids that flow around the connective and supporting tissues in the body. Called "ground" or "cement" substances, they provide strength and support to the body's tissues, including your skin.

They are composed of Glycosaminoglycans (GAGs), which attract approximately 60 – 70% water. Two of the most important GAGs are Hyaluronic acid (HA), which can attract 1,000 to 8,000 times its volume of water, and chondroitin sulfate. These two substances are the body's natural moisturizers and are essential for keeping the connective tissues hydrated. Water gives our tissues a spring-like ability, allowing them to return to their shape and withstand stress.[13]

As we age, we produce less GAG and HA, and that "stuff" around your cells becomes filled with more fibers than water. These fibers then form cross-links that bind to each other, making your tissues stiffer and less elastic. This cross-linking blocks the transport of nutrients into your cells and obstructs the removal of waste. Toxins and waste can then become trapped within your matrix making it harder for toxins to be released causing cellular weakness. In order to protect your vital organs, this extra toxicity will now cause your body to plump up the fat stores with these toxins. You end up with more fat on your body, feeling stiff and less flexible. Your connective tissue becomes dry and brittle, loses its elasticity and becomes weakened. The net result? *Cellulite and aging.*

Two keys to keeping your matrix hydrated and less rigid
There are two simple things—hydrate well and exercise. I can't emphasize enough the importance of regular movement like yoga, rebounding, and Pilates. When you compress your tissues with exercise, it can temporarily change the ground substance from gel to fluid, allowing the toxins and wastes to flow out of your matrix. Furthermore, when you exercise, it increases your blood supply and actually brings to your matrix all those good nutrients you have been mindfully consuming.

Cellulite is a result of leading a sedentary lifestyle. When you stop exercising regularly, the results can be very detrimental to your health in so many ways.

THE ROLE OF ESTROGEN

Proper function of the human body's systems is maintained by the careful output of hormones—one of the most notable being estrogen. Estrogen does not only control sex characteristics, it increases metabolic rate, and regulates blood viscosity and reduces LDL cholesterol in the blood. Two of the most vital roles estrogen plays in both males and females are the development and strengthening of the skin and other connective tissues, such as collagen. Estrogen maintains the proper activity of the cells and organs, such as the liver, gallbladder and adrenals, by regulating fat metabolism and its storage and use. This hormone is also largely responsible for how fat is dispersed under the skin.[14]

When estrogen, progesterone and testosterone levels are in balance the collagen "mesh" in the skin is strong and dense enough that any sub-dermal fatty deposits are contained. However, when the body falls into an estrogen-dominant state, the development of those visible fatty deposits, commonly known as cellulite, begins. Stress, especially chronic stress, contributes to the development of excess fatty deposits by taxing the adrenals and thyroid hormones. The adrenals and thyroid, along with other things, control the metabolism and use of excess fat.[15] When the body releases estrogen into the bloodstream, fluid begins to build in adipose (fatty) tissue underneath the skin. This sub-dermal layer of fat is not used by the body for energy production, except in times of dire need. It is mostly relied upon as a protective "pad" around bones and organs. The storage of excess fat around the hips and thighs also increases as the body acts to conserve enough for pregnancy and lactation in women. This is why many women first notice excess fat stores after childbirth or when taking the birth control pill.

Estrogen (in both genders) is also produced in larger quantities under times of stress, whether physical or mental, as a method of developing enough fat stores for the body to use in times of famine or other needs.

Estrogen is also responsible for weakening the connective tissue, known as septa, in order to accommodate growth during pregnancy and childbirth. Excess estrogen in the bloodstream also triggers the production of the hormone relaxin by the ovaries and breasts (in women) and the prostate (in men). Relaxin inhibits the production of collagen and further softens existing connective tissue. This action ensures both proper menstrual activity and sperm motility. In the highly hormonal final trimester of pregnancy, the levels of estrogen and relaxin are able to completely dissolve the collagen fibers. This is critical for widening the pubic bones, preparing the cervix for childbirth. However, less or weakened collagen in the skin allows for any fluid or fat swollen cells to push up, creating the characteristic "dimples" of cellulite.

Estrogen from external sources

Xenoestrogens are harmful, "external" estrogens that we absorb or ingest from artificial, external sources. They are commonly found in pesticides, plastics, detergents, and even perfumes. These chemicals are not always listed in ingredient lists, but include: parabens, phenoxyethanol, sodium laureth sulfate, PEG-100, phthalates polyethylene, Ceteareth-20, Oleth-2 and Oleth-10.

These compounds are toxic to the body. They can mimic the action of estrogen in our cells and alter our hormones.

Phytoestrogens are plant-based, naturally occurring estrogens that assist in normalizing levels of the hormone by binding to estrogen receptors. Once the estrogen receptors are occupied, external xenoestrogens have less of an ability to attach and impact the health the cell. It is beneficial to include plant products rich in phytoestrogens daily, because they bind to the open estrogen receptors and are much weaker in their hormonal effects. However, several recent studies have shown that certain phytoestrogens in supplement form can promote estrogen positive breast cancer under some circumstances. Therefore, it is always best to consume whole foods as opposed to supplements, where all the nutrients work synergistically together.

Cold-pressed oils made from seeds, nuts, and fruit (especially flax, sesame, and avocado) have been shown to have the greatest amount of phytoestrogens per serving. Never heat flax oil or sesame oil. You would be better off consuming ground flaxseeds, tahini (made from sesame seeds) and avocados. Beans, lentils, whole grains (such as millet and brown rice), seeds (including flax, quinoa, amaranth, alfalfa, fennel, anise, buckwheat, sesame, sunflower, and pumpkin), apples, pomegranates, sweet potatoes, yams, carrots, and dark green leafy vegetables are also rich in phytoestrogens.

Lymphatic activity and exercise

Less collagen in tissues is also responsible for a decrease in circulation and lymphatic activity. Daily exposure to toxins via the environment and diet is usually managed by the lymphatic system, which relies on external force to circulate lymph fluid. However, without a strong network of support, the vessels begin to become "floppy," leading to toxic build up, which causes excess fluid and fat retention. With daily aerobic exercise and regular stretching and massage, the blood vessels and muscles strengthen and the lymph is able to circulate more freely. Activity can include anything that increases heart rate for at least twenty minutes, including power walking, swimming, cross-country skiing, or skating.

Aerobic activity also assists in reducing the production of estrogen, as this hormone is both produced and stored in body fat. Maintaining a total body fat percentage between 18 – 28% in women and 12 – 20% in men is optimal for controlling excess estrogenic activity.

Nutrition to fight cellulite

To encourage the body's collagen production, adequate intake of several nutrients is required. These include lutein, hyaluronic acid, lycopene, vitamins A, C and E, sunflower lecithin, and essential fatty acids. To control estrogen levels, the body also relies on a high intake of vitamin B6, magnesium, and zinc in addition to natural, plant-based phytoestrogens found in food. Finally, support for the liver is necessary for eliminating excess hormones and other toxins in the body. Antioxidants and fiber prevent the build up of oxidizing material in the tissues.[16]

Blue, red or dark purple fruit and vegetables contain Anthocyanidins and Resveratrol found in blueberries, blackberries, black currants, cranberries, eggplant, tart cherries, pomegranates, plums, red cabbage, and red and black grapes. I know a lot of people think that drinking red wine is a good source of resveratrol, but unfortunately the alcohol dehydrates your skin, along with all the other damage it does. It is best to get resveratrol from organic red grapes. Anthocyanidins have been shown to protect collagen from the destructive effects of free radical damage.

- *Lutein* is found in dark green vegetables and is needed to metabolize proteins in order to increase the manufacture of collagen. Lutein has also been shown to promote the skin's ability to maintain hydration. Ten milligrams daily (4 oz. of spinach or 2 oz. of kale) is all you need.

- *Hyaluronic acid* (HA) is found in legumes and is important in maintaining collagen levels and flexibility. At least 2 tablespoons of legumes, or sprouted legumes, each day are required for adequate intake of this nutrient. Foods rich in magnesium, are essential for HA synthesis. Magnesium is found in all fruits and vegetables (especially dark leafy greens), carrots, raw nuts and seeds (especially sesame seeds and almonds), potatoes, whole grains, brown rice, avocados, bananas, apples, peaches, lima beans, and black-eyed peas. Starchy root vegetables, tubers, potatoes and sweet potatoes are also high in HA. Try eating some raw sweet potatoes to obtain even higher amounts of HA.

- *Lycopene*, vitamin A, vitamin C, vitamin E, and sulfur are all potent antioxidants and help your body produce collagen. Increasing your intake of red peppers, olives, cucumbers, celery, beets, tomatoes, squash, sweet potatoes, carrots, berries, and citrus will boost lycopene and the levels of vitamins A, C, and E in the body. Foods like garlic, onions and Brassica-family vegetables (brussels sprouts, broccoli, cabbage, and cauliflower), increase the body's sulfur levels.

These cruciferous vegetables may be easier to digest when lightly steamed, sautéed, juiced, baked, or made into soup.

A fresh juice containing cucumbers, celery, red bell peppers, cilantro, parsley, fennel, asparagus, kale, and other deep-green leafy veggies provides an ample supply of vitamins A, C and lycopene, as well as flavonoids, the essential fatty acids ALA (alpha-linolenic acid), and GLA (gamma-linolenic acid).

- *Lecithin* is a naturally occurring fat emulsifier and is critical to the body's cellular repair and growth. Adequate levels of lecithin improve the density and strength of the collagen network, effectively managing the appearance of cellulite. Sunflower lecithin, cauliflower, potatoes, spinach, tomatoes, and oranges are all good sources of lecithin.

Excess estrogen production has been strongly linked to dietary deficiencies in vitamin B6, zinc, and magnesium. Vitamin B6 and magnesium are responsible for detoxifying estrogen as it enters the liver. Zinc blocks the enzyme responsible for converting excess testosterone (common in women) into estrogen. Squash (especially winter varieties), beets, seeds (sunflower, sesame, and pumpkin) spinach, chard, legumes, and bananas are prime sources of these nutrients.

The liver must detoxify estrogen before it can be eliminated, and the liver is greatly affected when the amount of the hormone is high. Cruciferous vegetables (broccoli, cabbage, cauliflower) provide the necessary "push" towards the elimination pathway. Melons, pineapples, pears, grapes, berries, and citrus fruits also assist in this liver detoxification and are helpful in inhibiting excess estrogen production.

A diet rich in antioxidants supports the liver processes and minimizes free radical damage to collagen and skin cells. Did you know that most pesticides—fungicides and other chemical cocktails that are used on vegetables, fruits, and soy—not only raise the toxicity of the food, but also encourage estrogen dominance?

Studies on coffee consumption and estrogen have shown that women who drink four to five cups of coffee a day had a nearly 70% higher estrogen level during the early part of their menstrual cycle than women who drink less than one cup of coffee a day.

According to a Cornell University study, alcohol consumption in women is thought to affect the way estrogen is actually broken down and secreted by the body. Increased alcohol consumption can lead to a significant increase in the levels of estrogen, damaging the liver cells and interfering with other toxic eliminations.[17]

Detoxification and Its Positive Effects

"Detoxification" is a buzzword nowadays and it is displayed everywhere—from packages of herbal products to powerful nutritional regimens. You will hear it on the news as your favorite celebrity tells you about her latest cleansing routine. Your trainer will no doubt mention it, as you progress on your path towards healthy and youthful living. However, what most people don't realize is that detoxification is an ongoing natural process inside the body.

Every day, minute, and second of your life, there is a delicate balance of building and destroying going on within and around each of your cells. As we build, create and use energy, we generate waste products that must be eliminated. Without this elimination process, we would drown in our own waste, first at the cellular level, but eventually our whole organism would suffocate, and death would result.

Now don't panic, you don't have to monitor all these life-sustaining processes—that's not your job. Your job is to make sure you provide your body and mind with plenty of nutritionally dense food, pure water and fresh air. Rest, sleep, and relaxing activities help us recover after hard work. The idea of relaxation is very close to detoxification. In essence, when you truly relax, you release toxic energy, nerve impulses, and thoughts that are burdening your body and mind, hindering the healing process or the maintenance of a healthy lifestyle.

*Detoxification is about getting rid of substances that
are not useful for us.*

Most people talk about detoxification in glamorous terms, as if it was the easiest thing to do. Let me assure you that getting rid of anything is not easy. Saying "no" to items we are accustomed to eating, drinking, and thinking about presents us with hurdles we must overcome. It is not easy to say no to a slice of double fudge cake or your mom's unforgettable pie with a smile.

When it comes to your cellulite, perhaps you are thinking more in terms of temporary measures, or you may be ready for completely clearing your path to cellulite-free living. Whatever your goal is, detoxification is a must.

Your skin is an eliminative organ

Detoxification happens through our skin via perspiration. As a result, when toxins come out, acne, boils, recurring eczema, and psoriasis may appear. These are symptoms of toxicity, and some of them are almost impossible to heal using current medical treatments. Why are they so difficult to heal? Our popular concept of "healing" too often means covering up the symptoms with creams or lotions or ingesting very powerful pharmaceutical compounds that have serious side effects. Even then they may not do the job, because without addressing the real root causes and internal toxins, the rash or problems will keep recurring. Instead of focusing on the symptom, we need to look at the causes and the hints the body is giving us. It is oftentimes not about adding some pill, potion, vitamin supplement, or medicine, but rather eliminating dietary excesses and making changes to our lifestyle in order to restore our health. Unfortunately, most of us are looking for health in the wrong places.

A rash is a very important detoxification process that should be viewed as a good sign—the body is saying goodbye to poisons. The same goes for the dimpled, orange-peel-looking, sagging or folding skin that seems to just appear from nowhere.

Our bodies are designed to constantly remove toxins from our cells. Most of the toxins are broken down by our liver and then eliminated via our kidneys, colon, skin, lungs, and mucus linings in our nose and ears. When there is an excess amount of toxins our body increases its output, but in order to preserve our health, it stores the excess toxins into pockets of subcutaneous fat, protecting the important organs that keep you alive.

Your liver is an eliminative organ
Your liver is your second largest eliminative organ, after your skin. It works day and night to produce enzymes made from proteins to help neutralize the toxic parts of our lives. It pays to look after your liver by eating well, drinking enough clean water, and tending to your emotions in a caring and nurturing way. Anger and frustration are very powerful emotions that trigger the liver into producing chemical compounds that are harmful. It is easy to see that living with balanced emotions will also speed up any healing, and rejuvenate the look and feel of your skin.

Your colon is an eliminative organ
The next important avenue of detoxification is the colon, where we release the majority of the fibers we take in. Although we cannot assimilate fiber, we must have fibrous foods to help us escort the waste products from our stomach, small intestine and large intestine. When we eat foods with no fiber, like cheese, eggs, meat, fish, and bread made with white flour, we will experience less than optimal elimination for the next few days. This can then lead to headaches and irritability, with others and ourselves.

We need to be eating fiber every day for healthy detoxification. If you are eating a lot of fruits and vegetables you are getting all the fiber your body needs. Always make sure to increase your water consumption as you increase your fiber.

Your lungs are an eliminative organ
Detoxification through the lungs is both the easiest and hardest to control. If we take shallow and/or fast breaths, the exchange of clean air and waste is inefficient and slow. This can lead to illnesses of the lungs, throat, mouth, and sinus cavities of the face. The all too common headache is also a sign of improper breathing. Sign up for yoga classes where they offer Pranayama, and you will never take your breath for granted.

Your kidneys are an eliminative organ
Your kidneys work hard filtering your blood supply and passing all the undesirables to the bladder for elimination. Pay attention to nagging and unexplained backaches and urinary problems. Your kidneys could be in trouble. Clean, filtered water in ample quantity every day will help your kidneys function.

Now that you have a better understanding of what detoxification is and why you need it, let's talk about those fatty deposits and how to keep them away. Interestingly, those deposits are a safety mechanism of your body.

When you eat or drink nutrient deficient, chemical laden, dehydrating substances your tissues can become dry, brittle, and weak. Your body, in its infinite wisdom, is able to do a marvelous job of protecting your organs by buffering any harsh acids that could damage your organs and hinder the life sustaining processes in your system. Your amazing body is constantly at work gathering up and removing toxins from your cells. If your eliminative organs cannot keep up, then your body stores toxins in your fat tissue, tucking them as far away as possible from your organs and glands. Fatty deposits are first formed under your skin, as far as possible from your heart, lungs and bloodstream. In the short term, these fatty deposits are your savior. Your body has stashed away the toxic substances in these pockets of fat. Cellulite occurs as a result of these fat deposits being pushed through layers of the weakened connective tissue under your skin.

To treat cellulite successfully, you must help your body to eliminate toxins to reduce those fatty deposits, while strengthening your connective tissues. You can apply a local castor oil pack on your liver or on your buttocks to improve circulation. The long-range plan has to be a daily, healthy diet of green vegetables, root vegetables, fresh fruits, and pure water. Sufficient exercise that includes deep breathing will relax the body and mind and stimulate the lymphatic drainage of all waste products throughout the body.

– 12 –

The Detoxification Process

"Health is a matter of choice, not a mystery of chance."
~ Aristotle

It is important to remember that today we are all surrounded by toxic chemicals that find their way into our bodies through the air we breathe, the food we eat, and the water we drink. In addition to these external toxins, the body continuously produces internal toxins through normal metabolic processes such as digestion and other cellular activities. This means the process of detoxification is a normal and necessary activity that the body continuously engages in. It eliminates or neutralizes toxins through the colon, liver, kidneys, lungs, lymph, and skin.

The body is always striving to establish balance or homeostasis. This balance is disturbed when we feed ourselves more than we can utilize and ingest substances that are toxic to the body. If our system cannot tolerate the excess wastes, the body will reabsorb them. This then raises the overall toxicity level, and that can lead to disease. The body handles toxins by either neutralizing, transforming, eliminating, or storing them.

If these toxins cannot be eliminated or transformed, they can destroy enzymes, stagnate in the tissues and interfere with circulation, which results in a decreased availability of nutrients to cells. Toxins can also interact with hormones, causing imbalances. All these factors contribute to the formation of cellulite in the body.

Cleansing and elimination are very important pieces of the nutritional therapy puzzle. The others are rebuilding through vegetable juicing and increasing the consumption of vegetables, dark leafy greens, and fruit. This will help with balancing the mineral ratios, hydration and the look of your skin. Don't forget to include meditation and yoga, which are necessary on an emotional and spiritual level.

The body has a daily elimination cycle, carried out mostly during the night and early morning, up until breakfast. However, if we eat foods containing unhealthy fats, meats, dairy products, refined foods, and chemical preservatives, we slow down the process. This makes detoxification even more crucial to staying healthy. When consuming meat, you are also consuming all the chemicals that were injected into the animal, that have accumulated in the animal's fatty tissue, and will end up in the tissues of your body.

The problem

If the body has been weakened through over-stimulation, overeating or sleep deprivation, the body's natural cleansing process can become overloaded. The toxins could accumulate in your lymph nodes and can even get into your bloodstream, which can create diseases. To keep the blood as pure as possible, the body will protect itself by dumping these toxins into the surrounding tissues. Toxins suffocate your cells and deprive them of the nutrients, water and oxygen they require.

It should now be easy to see how the choices we make every day impact our cellular health. If we want vibrant good health and radiant glowing skin, then we must make changes in our diet and lifestyle choices to reduce the intake of toxins and improve elimination.

The solution
The first step is to simplify your diet. Cut out all the foods that are unhealthy for you. Don't eat packaged, refined or deep fried foods and avoid fatty meats or luncheon meats. Avoid sugar, alcohol, caffeine, artificial sweeteners, dairy fats, milk, processed cheese, preservatives, soft drinks, potato chips, and fast foods. Limit your consumption of wheat (gluten) and soy. Cut out all vegetable oils like sunflower, canola, and peanut oil. Avoid over-the-counter medications, tobacco, and crash diets.

Correct any imbalances that are caused by chronic stress, shallow breathing, constipation, over-eating, lack of sleep, and lack of movement from sitting all day. The word emotion contains the word motion, to help balance your mood, so start exercising. Start walking and incorporating yoga, rebounding, or Pilates. Practice deep breathing, meditation, and start relaxing. Take up activities that please your heart as opposed to only doing things to please others. Take baths in minerals like Epsom salts to help your circulation.

Replace tap water with filtered or distilled water and add 1 teaspoon of greens powder or liquid chlorophyll, wheat grass juice, or barley grass.

Make healthier food choices: fresh fruits, avocados, green leafy vegetables, root vegetables (beets, potatoes, sweet potatoes, squash), legumes, whole grains (quinoa, millet), and buckwheat. Non-sweet fruits (tomatoes, cucumbers), citrus, berries, and sweeter fruits are really healthy choices.

Raw (not roasted) unsalted nuts and seeds can provide an ample amount of protein and healthy fat. Refrigerate or freeze them to prevent them from going rancid. Avoid buying them from bulk bins, which may contain rancid fats and mold. One handful of raw nuts is a serving.

Choose healthy oils: coconut oil is safe for cooking. The fats that should never be heated are: olive oil, avocado oil, flaxseed oil and hemp oil, as these oils are extremely vulnerable to heat, light, and air.

Proper elimination is important; having more than one bowel movement per day is necessary. Far Infrared sauna treatments will help to eliminate toxins through sweating. Rebounding at least twice per day will get the lymphatic system moving.

One of the first steps in reducing the fatty deposits is correcting your mineral balance by consuming nutrient dense food. This will help to reduce your cravings, so you can make healthier choices and begin to lose excess fat. Reducing body fat will also reduce any debris that has built up in your body over the years from dietary and environmental toxins. Drinking lots of pure water and increasing your fiber intake by including more fruits, vegetables, and greens in your diet are steps in the detoxification process.

Have a nutrient-rich cleanse day every week. On that day plan to rest and not exercise. Restorative or yin yoga and gentle stretching is encouraged. Drink fresh vegetable juices throughout the day and evening or eat fresh fruit all day. Drink plenty of water and rest when needed.

Overeating can be very detrimental, forcing your digestive organs to work overtime hindering your overall health. A cleanse day allows the body to do its "internal house cleaning," giving your digestive organs a much needed rest.

Vegetable juices are full of vitamins and minerals. Fruit is astringent and helpful in drawing out toxins. As a result, the body begins to break up the fatty deposits. Obesity is almost always associated with toxicity. The extra body fat contains toxins and creates inflammation in the body. During fat loss, we release toxins and need to make sure we drink enough filtered or distilled water throughout the day to flush them out. It is very important to take in fiber-rich foods and antioxidant nutrients like vitamins A, C, E, beta-carotene, selenium, and zinc. You can find them naturally in fresh vegetables, fruits, raw nuts and seeds.

Let go of what no longer serves you, in all aspects of your life. Most people have a natural tendency to hold onto old eating patterns, even after they have learned these patterns are harmful and not nourishing. This only leads to congestion and feeling stuck. Start choosing foods that make you feel vitalized and clear, not lethargic and stressed.

Less is more. As we get older, we require less food in general. To cut down on the quantity of food, start to consume more nutrient dense and less calorie dense foods. Nutrient dense foods include green leafy vegetables, sprouts, fruits, legumes, whole gluten-free grains, and small amounts of raw nuts and seeds. They are wholesome and full of nutrients as found in nature, in contrast to foods that come in boxes or are available at the drive-thru. Calorie dense foods are those that contain a large amount of calories in relation to their portion size, with little or no nutritional value. Food becomes calorie dense when it is refined and processed with added fat, sodium, sugar and preservatives to increase shelf life and improve taste. Calorie dense foods that have little or no nutritional value include donuts, ice cream, potato chips, candy, soft drinks, sugary cereals, puddings, and most store bought baked goods and boxed cookies. These foods rob you of nutrients in order to be metabolized and leave you feeling unsatisfied and still hungry.

Mental detoxification is also important. Cleansing your mind of negative thoughts and learning to accept and love yourself unconditionally is essential to good health.

Detoxification helps us uncover any residual emotions we may have tucked away or swept under the carpet. The process of releasing physical toxins allows these unacknowledged emotions to rise to the surface for us to tend to by first understanding, feeling and then accepting them. We must then release them and move on. Otherwise we will feel limited or stuck, unable to move forward in our lives. Our thoughts and perceptions can keep us feeling enslaved. Pressures and self-imposed limits are in our mind. To be free of them we must first understand them. We must become aware of the things that enslave us on a subconscious level. We are all slaves to something in our lives, whether it's a food or substance addiction, or internal expectations of how things and people around us should be. We have to let go and realize that we can achieve anything we set out to do. True freedom has to do with your state of mind.

– 13 –

Your Daily Detoxifying Routine

Focusing on daily detoxification will help to increase energy, reduce cellulite, and rejuvenate your skin. Not only will your skin thank you, so will your immune system, metabolism, along with your mood and energy levels. Detoxes can leave you feeling lighter and happier, rejuvenated and ready to take on the world!

Hydrate

First thing in the morning, drink a large glass of room temperature filtered water. Then you can prepare a mixture consisting of three liters of purified water and a greens powder, liquid chlorophyll or fresh lemon to drink throughout the day. The best greens powders are either Athletic greens or Barley Max, which are sold online. You can also juice fresh wheatgrass, which is high in chlorophyll. The idea is to make sure you are drinking a lot of water with greens, especially at the beginning. This will give your body the vitamins, minerals, and enzymes it needs to help balance, cleanse, and begin to heal.

Exfoliate

In the morning before you shower or bathe, you can exfoliate or dry brush your body. Dry brushing with a long handled brush made with natural bristles helps to tighten your skin and increases blood flow and helps the lymphatic system release toxins.

Rebounding
Bounce on a rebounder for at least fifteen minutes. A rebounder is a small, circular mini-trampoline that is easy to bounce on. Invest in a good rebounder, with either bungee cord structure or wire coil springs. Some rebounders come with a stability bar, so you can hold on while you bounce. Rebounding will benefit lymphatic circulation to help remove toxins. It helps to circulate more oxygen to the tissues and helps with cellulite reduction. (*See page 105.*)

Juice for breakfast
Drink a large fresh vegetable juice or have a fruit smoothie for breakfast. Continue having fresh juices all day or eat a light lunch consisting of a homemade vegetable soup with some quinoa or a sweet potato stew. For more ideas, please see the meal planning guide in chapter 17.

Relax
We commonly hold on to stress in our muscles and in the tissues near our skin. Try to arrange your daily schedule so that you are not rushing around stressed. Go outside for a gentle walk in the fresh air or sit quietly and meditate to relax your muscles. Start your day with a 15-minute meditation and some gentle yoga. Remind yourself to breathe and trust in yourself and everything that is happening in your life. You can then truly let go, relax and feel that everything is going to work out exactly as it should.

Far infrared sauna therapy
If available, infrared sauna therapy helps to reduce cellulite, by increasing our metabolism to burn fat and decongesting our lymph system by eliminating toxins. Far infrared rays penetrate beneath our skin and speed up metabolic exchanges between cells and elevate our temperature. Our body reacts to infrared rays by dilating blood

vessels and thus improving circulation. With more effective circulation, oxygen and nutrients are carried more efficiently to the cells.

Throughout the day

Once again, hydration is really important to help the kidneys more effectively filter out the toxins that have been mobilized by dry brushing, rebounding and the reduction in the amount of processed food you have consumed. Keep drinking filtered water in small increments. Slower is better and more effective.

Castor oil packs

You can place a castor oil pack on the areas of your body that have cellulite. Preparing a castor oil pack is very simple:

1. Saturate a 10" x 10" flannel sheet with Palma Christi filtered castor oil and place it on the area to be treated.
2. You can add the benefit of heat by covering the soaked flannel with a plastic bag and placing a hot-water bottle or heating pad on top.

This will help disperse the toxins that have been mobilized by all the healthy changes you are making.

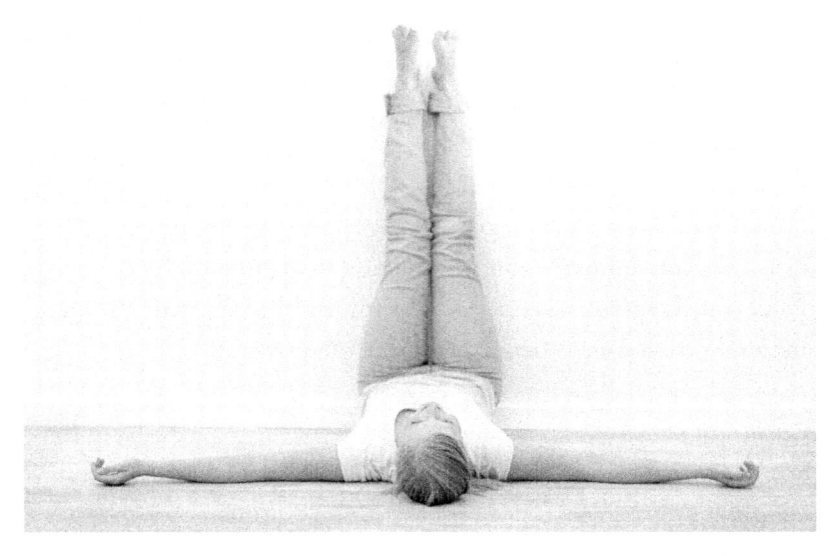

Vipariti Karani (Wall Leg Pose)

Movement and stretching
It is really helpful to practice some of the gentle yoga routines you will find in this book, especially Vipariti Karani (waterfall pose) and other longer held, forward stretches.

Your next meal
Make sure your next meal is a nutritious meal from the meal planning guide in chapter 17. A fresh vegetable juice or a fruit smoothie is the fastest acting meal replacement, which provides immediate nutrition but requires no digestion. This will allow your body to focus on detoxifying rather than on the work of digestion.

The next day
Have an Epsom salt bath then get back to rebounding and exercising.

- 14 -

Exercise and the Lymphatic System

Most people are not aware of how important it is to exercise for just thirty minutes every day. Many of us, after sitting at a desk all day, drive home in traffic and end up slouched on the couch. Then later, exhausted, we finally go to bed. The next day, the same process repeats itself. Some people may argue that walking to the car or to the bus stop, preparing food, doing dishes, or mowing the lawn is plenty of movement for them. However, this will not promote healthy living for the long run.

We have lymphatic vessels in our bodies, which are a mesh-like network of tubes, filled with lymph fluid. This extra-cellular fluid flows only one way, removing excess fluid, waste, debris, dead blood cells, pathogens, cancer cells, and toxins from our cells and tissues. Our lymphatic system has the very important role of mopping up (cleaning) all that is not needed.

The lymphatic system also works with your circulatory system to deliver nutrients, oxygen and hormones from the blood to the cells that make up your body tissues. More importantly, your lymphatic system aids your immune system in destroying pathogens and filtering waste so that the lymph can be safely returned to the circulatory system.

Your blood is pumped by your heart, circulates throughout your body and is cleansed and filtered by your kidneys. Your lymphatic system, however, does not have a pump to aid in its flow; instead this system is designed so that movements of your muscles stimulate the flow of lymph into the capillaries. Your lymph flows only one way, traveling from your extremities (feet and hands) and upward through the body towards your neck. As it travels through the body lymph passes through lymph nodes, where it is filtered. At the base of your neck, the lymph enters the subclavian vein and once again becomes plasma in your bloodstream.

The average human body has between six and seven hundred lymph nodes, where the lymph is filtered before it can be returned to the circulatory system. Your lymph nodes can increase or decrease in size throughout your life but any nodes that have been damaged or destroyed will not regenerate.

Within each lymph node specialized white blood cells called lymphocytes kill any pathogens that may be present. This can cause swelling, commonly known as swollen glands. Lymph nodes also trap cancer cells and slow the spread of the cancer, until they are overwhelmed by it.

Knowing the important role your lymph plays will make it easier to understand the importance of movement and exercise. The movements of your muscles stimulate the flow of the lymph into the capillaries. Without exercise, your lymph system can become very sluggish. Lymphatic stagnation is one of the most commonly overlooked causes of cellulite and edema (an excess of watery fluid collecting in the cavities or tissues of the body).

A healthy lymphatic system will help to reduce cellulite, the orange-peel-like skin that forms when fluid distorts the cells in and around your fat, creating dimples in your skin.

WHAT IS THE BEST KIND OF EXERCISE TO HELP YOUR LYMPHATIC SYSTEM?

Yoga

You need to ensure your lymphatic system is healthy so it is able to remove excess fluid, waste, debris and toxins. The best exercises are those that allow the lymph to move forward toward the neck. Yoga is one of the safest and most effective exercises to perform this task. Look at any yoga posture and you'll understand. During a one-hour yoga session those postures provide the perfect drainage to all your lymph nodes.

What's more, the possibility of injury is minimal if you practice with a qualified teacher. Yoga is a very thorough exercise, where you benefit from consistent practice. Just a few months of regular yoga classes will rev up your system inside out.

Deep breathing

Deep breathing stimulates our lymphatic system and improves blood flow, aiding in the natural detoxification process. When you oxygenate your cells, expand your lungs, eliminate toxins and stress, you'll quickly notice how young and radiant your skin looks.

Rebounding

Second to yoga, rebounding is a fantastic lymph exercise. If done daily, it will do wonders for your whole body, including your lymphatic system. Each time you bounce up, the lymph fluid moves towards your limbs, and each time you land the lymph is forced towards the neck. Just ten minutes of rebounding is equivalent to thirty minutes of walking.

To run or not to run
Many people take up running as an all over exercise regime, not realizing the minuscule injuries that occur daily to the bones of the feet, ankle, shin, knees, and hips. These hair-like fractures accumulate into imbalances, pushing the runner into further injuries. After a few years or decades, another hip or knee surgery is needed. Meanwhile, pain is constant and exercise becomes almost impossible to continue.

Swimming
Swimming is good, especially if you can swim in the ocean or a lake, but there is no lymphatic drainage.

Walking
Brisk walking with your arms moving is helpful for your lymphatic system. There are so many lymph nodes in the upper body, armpits, neck, and shoulders that moving your arms is important. A wonderful walk in the fresh air is refreshing and healthy, and is a great way to take a break and reduce stress.

Make exercise a daily routine. To stay on track with exercise, write how you feel in a journal. I use food and mood journals in my practice to help clients become aware of patterns. Journaling your exercise routine is helpful to keep you on track. Some doubts, frustration, boredom and tiredness may set in, which also should be written down. Looking back at earlier entries in the journal will help overcome any laziness or doubt that sets in, so you can continue on your path to diminished cellulite, less body fat, and overall better health and vitality.

– 15 –

Yoga Routines for Cellulite Reduction

Yoga trains the body and mind for skillful living. Yoga postures harness the abilities of the body, control the busy mind and leave you refreshed and strong. Here are some good yoga sequences you might enjoy for a healthy body.

SEQUENCE 1

1. **Deep breathing** for two minutes. Sitting or standing, fill your lungs to capacity by breathing in through your nose and out through your open mouth with a soft 'ha' sound.

2. **Sun salutations** — Three sets (*Follow illustrations on page 108*).
   a) Stand tall with your hands in prayer position in front of your heart.
   b) Lift your arms straight above your head. Look up as you inhale.
   c) Exhale through your mouth; bend forward and touch the floor. Bend your knees or keep them straight. Relax your head, neck and spine. This is Forward Fold.
   d) Inhale and step back with your right leg, knee on the floor, top of the foot flat on the mat. Look up. Lift your trunk, arms over your head, palms facing one another, head gently back.

This is the Crescent Moon pose. Don't strain.

e) Exhale and place your hands on the floor in front of your left foot; step your left leg back. Either stay on your knees or come up into a high plank position with your body straight and parallel to the floor. Keep your body and legs strong.

f) Retain your breath, then exhale and bend your arms; lower your body down to 1 inch from the mat. Stay strong.

g) Lie on your belly; inhale; press your hands into the mat under your shoulders and lift your upper body up, stretching back into a Cobra pose. Keep your hips on the mat.

h) Exhale; lift up into a sharp inverted V or Downward Facing Dog, hips to the ceiling, legs straight, heels pressing into the mat, arms and chest straight.

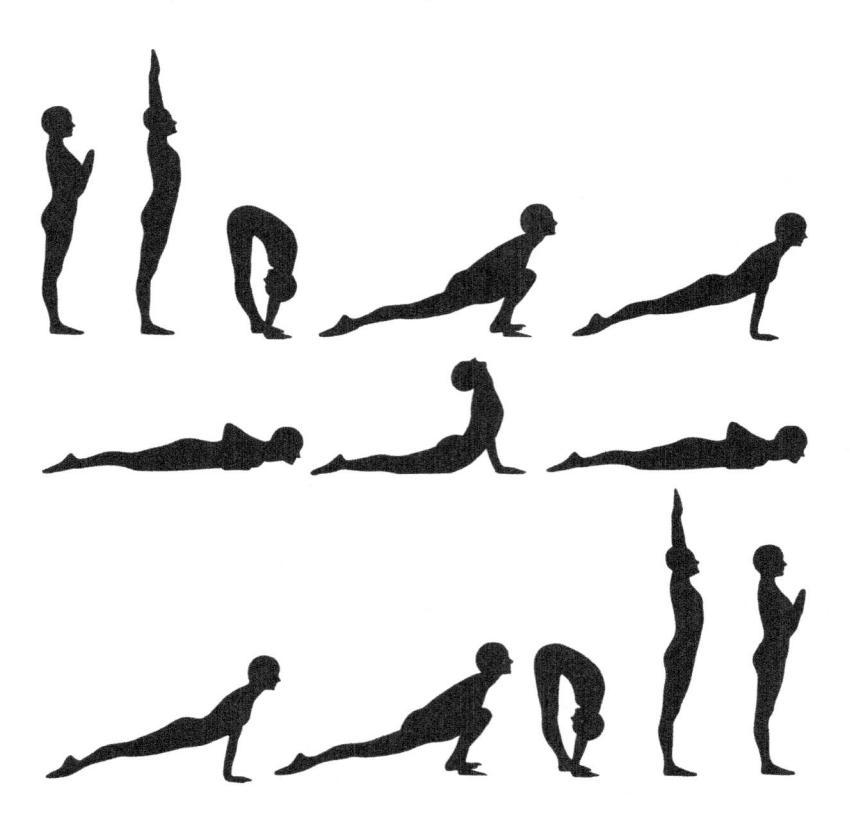

i) Inhale; extend the right leg up towards the sky; open up the hip on the right side, then as you exhale, swing the leg forward and bring your foot down in between your hands, left knee on the floor.
j) Inhale; lift your trunk and arms up, arch gently back repeating the Crescent Moon pose again.
k) Exhale; hands to mat, step forward with the left leg, both feet between the hands. Hang there upside down. Forward Fold again.
l) Inhale; stand up, arms above your head.

Repeat steps 'b' to 'k' alternating the leading leg from right to left and then right again until you have finished three sets.

By the time you are done, you should have a light sweat or at least be feeling warm.

3. **Standing side stretch**

   Stand tall, then jump the legs open 4 to 5 feet apart. Extend arms at shoulder height. Turn your right foot out to a 90 degree angle; turn in your left foot to a 20 degree angle. Bend your right knee as far as you can, leaning into it while keeping your body straight. Don't strain.

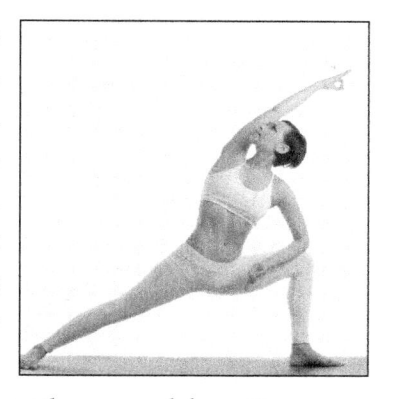

   It is important to keep your breath even and deep. Keep your mind focused and steady. Hold this pose for five long breaths. Stretch your left arm over your left ear as you lower the right arm and right hand toward the mat. Your trunk will be leaning towards the right side. Lengthen the side, breathe evenly. Keep your chest turning towards the sky.

Keep your arms strong. Keep your right leg at the right angle. Don't strain. Stay for five deep breaths, come up. Repeat on the other side.

4. **Bound angle stretch**

   Sit on the mat; bring the bottoms of your feet together very close to your groin. Sit tall, spine erect. Grab your feet with both hands and hinging from your hips, gently lean forward as far as you comfortably can. Go slowly; go deeply, but don't strain. Stay for five deep, long breaths. On an exhale, reach forward with your arms at the end of the pose to go even deeper, if you can.

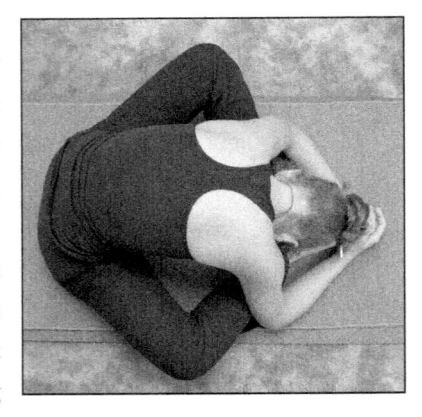

5. **Supine hero pose**

   From the bound angle pose previously described, come out by sitting up tall again.

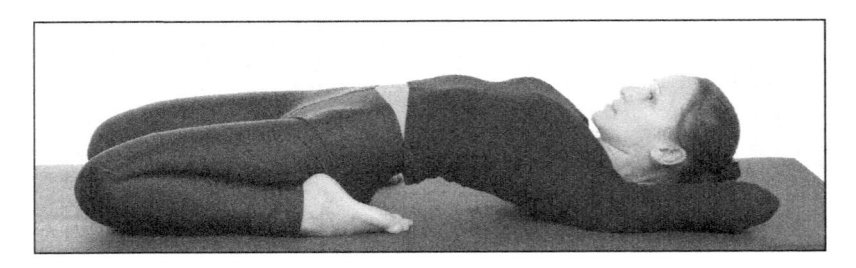

   Bring your legs beside your hips, one at a time, very close to the side of the buttocks, toes slightly turning toward your hips. Bring your knees together, as close as possible. Don't force it. Once you feel relaxed and somewhat comfortable in the pose, slowly lean back onto your elbows, one at a time, then lower your back onto the floor. Breathe deeply. Stop if your knees hurt sharply, or your ankles scream for attention. Both will pass, but it is better to be gradual than forceful. It may take you days, weeks, even months of daily practice before you can lie down comfortably in this pose. Keep practicing. It is a wonderful pose for the legs, hips and even for digestion.

After five long deep breaths on the floor, sit up using your arms. Rescue the legs by straightening them; lie on your back for thirty seconds to enjoy the after effects of blood rushing into the previously stretched regions of the legs. You will feel a surge of energy rushing through your whole body!

6. **Twist**

Sit with your legs in front, straight. Cross your right foot over your left leg. Bend the left leg and bring the left foot close to the side of the body. The right foot is flat, close to the left knee on the floor. Lift the left arm up; open up your rib cage; turn toward the right side; bring the left arm down on the outside of the right leg; reach for the left knee; grab it and turn the torso to the right, looking over the right shoulder. Keep it slow, feeling your way into the twist. Forcing it may result in impaired breathing, bruised ribs and an overall unhappy yogi. Once you have reached your maximum twist, stay there, smile, and count five deep breaths.

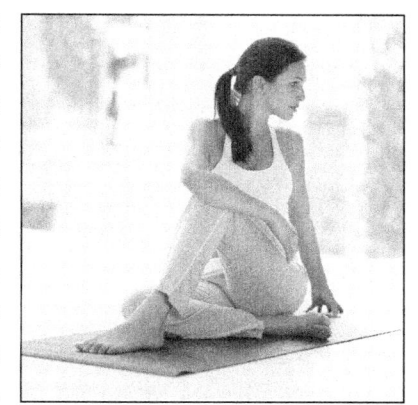

Change sides, changing leg and arm positions.

7. **Savasana**

   The final relaxation is the most important pose of any yoga practice. Without this final rest, it is like making a soup, tasting it but never actually getting to enjoy a whole bowl. You need to master the art of relaxation. One simple way is to make sure nothing is distracting you. Lie down on your mat and cover yourself with a blanket to further relax. Let go of your arms, legs, back, and head. Close your eyes and breathe deeply. As you relax, your breath will quiet down and then your brain quiets down. You may even fall asleep. A ten-minute nap will not hurt anyone. Set a timer if you must. It is better to relax for five minutes with a timer, than worry about falling asleep, and struggle to stay relaxed on the floor for twenty minutes.

SEQUENCE 2

1. As with Sequence 1, begin with a deep breathing exercise, for two minutes. Sitting or standing, fill your lungs to capacity by breathing in through your nose and out through your open mouth with a soft "ha" sound.

2. **Fierce pose**

   Lift your arms over your head, interlock all fingers and straighten your arms with your biceps to your ears. Hold the pose steady. Don't force the shoulders. Breathe smoothly. Slowly bend your knees, press them together throughout, until you reach a semi-sitting position. This is a challenging pose. Keep your chest lifting, arms lifting, all the while still sitting down. Hold for five breaths. Then gently twist to the right and bring the left elbow to the outside of the right thigh. Sit lower. Twist the body gently. Don't strain.

Inhale, release and fold forward with your hands to the mat. Keep the legs straight or slightly bent, bring the arms behind the back and interlace your fingers while squeezing your shoulder blades together. Lift your arms over your head. Two long breaths will do fine. Inhale and bring your arms in front of your body and interlock your fingers again stretching your arms over your head and lifting your torso up, but still sitting down as before. Twist to the other side. Five breaths there, too. Once done, fold again forward and bring the arms behind the back and pull the arms over the head gently. Inhale and stand up and shake it out.

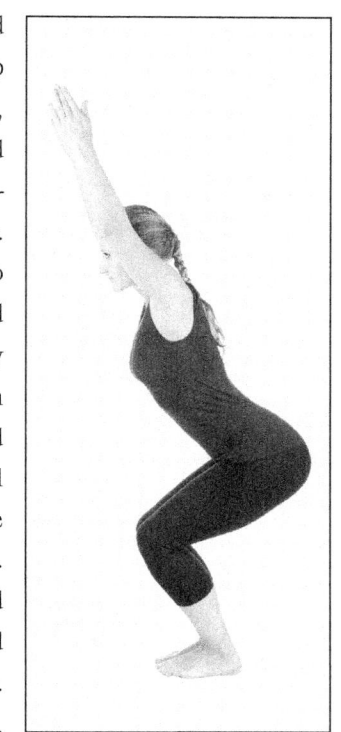

3. **Standing transverse triangle**

    Stand with legs apart and arms extended at shoulder height. To make it challenging for the inner thighs, spread the legs more. Inhale and suck the belly in, bend forward at the hips slowly with straight legs and straight back. Once close to the floor, grab your feet or place your hands on your mat between your legs. Inhale. Lift your head a bit, straighten the spine more and exhale. Keep folding forward more, until your head touches the floor. Feel your legs and back stretching.

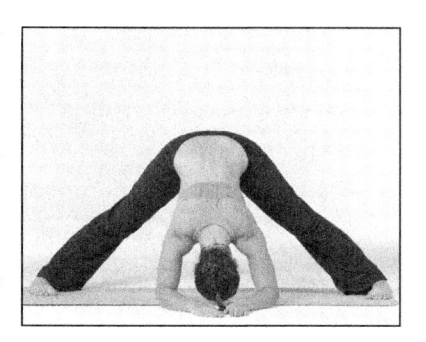

4. **Standing leg splits**

   Next inhale stand up and turn to the left. Lower the right knee onto the mat and try to keep the left leg straight for half splits. With hands on the floor beside your leg, lengthen forward, increasing the stretch sensitively, never forcing it. Breathe through your nose evenly and deeply. Hold the stretch for five breaths. Inhale, come up and lift the back knee, then turn to the other side and repeat.

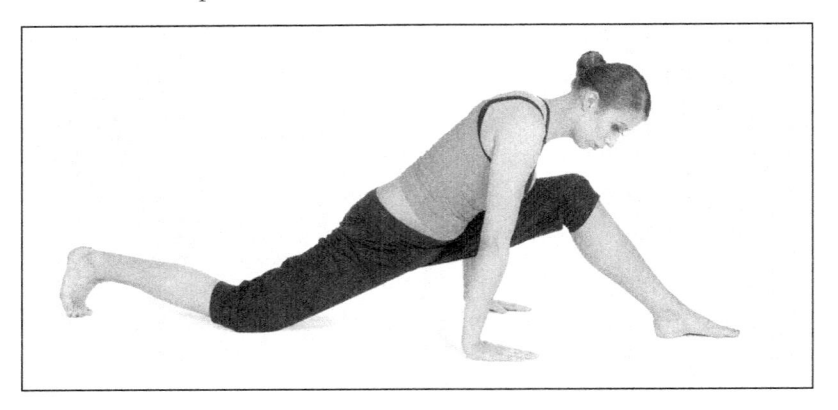

5. **Eagle pose**

   Stand tall. Inhale with arms over the head. As you exhale, twist your arms in front of your chest, so elbows and wrists cross. Place palms together or grab the hands with a strong grip. Pull the arms down to open up the upper back and shoulders. Now, lift your right leg up and cross over the left thigh in a nice tight crossing, then hook your toes behind the left calf muscles. This should bring a strong sensation as the muscles along the shin and the side of the thighs stretch.

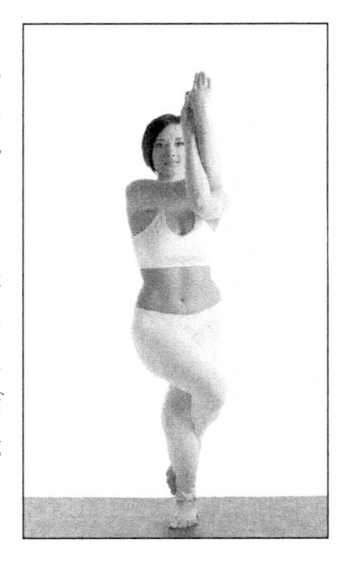

Sit down more; feel the side hips stretch. This pose is excellent for a stretch of all those areas that are almost impossible to stretch otherwise.

Release after five deep breaths, then repeat with the opposite configuration: left arm under the right arm, left leg over the right leg.

6. **Bridge pose**

Lie down with your arms long beside your body. Bring your feet close to your buttocks. Feet flat. Inhale and lift your hips then your spine slowly and gradually, all the way up. Then stop and exhale while slowly lowering the spine and your hips down. Repeat three times. Once more, inhale and lift all the way up and hold while you bring your hands to your buttocks, fingers towards your legs and support your lower back. Stay here feeling the tremendous stretch for the front of the body. Feel your legs, hips, pubic bone area, and lower abdomen, all nicely stretching with your lower back and arms strengthening. This is a fantastic pose to strengthen your back, and sculpt the thighs. Lower your body down and rest after five deep breaths.

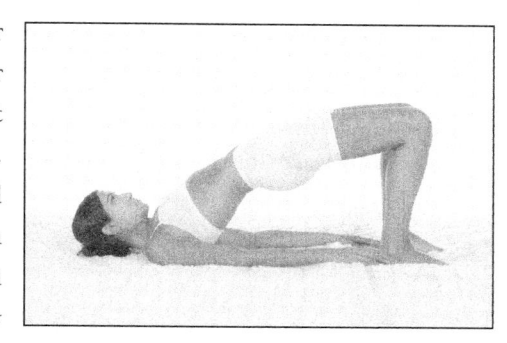

7. **Forward stretch**

Simple but very powerful, this is one of the most basic postures, which works wonders for the legs and back, as well as the abdominal region. Exercise with caution and do not bounce back and forth. Hold the stretch steadily and you will no doubt find this pose very effective on many areas.

Sit on the floor with straight legs in front and hands beside your buttocks. Press your fingertips down to the floor as you start gently pushing down the torso forward towards the legs. Once you have reached your maximum, stop pushing with the hands and reach forward towards the toes, and grab them if you can. If not, grab your ankles or lower legs. Gently pull forward and relax your head and breathe evenly. Do not strain. Five deep breaths will suffice. Relax.

8. **Vipariti Karani**

   The pose that does absolute marvels to the legs and visible veins or cellulite is this gentle inversion, which is safe for everyone, unless you are pregnant.

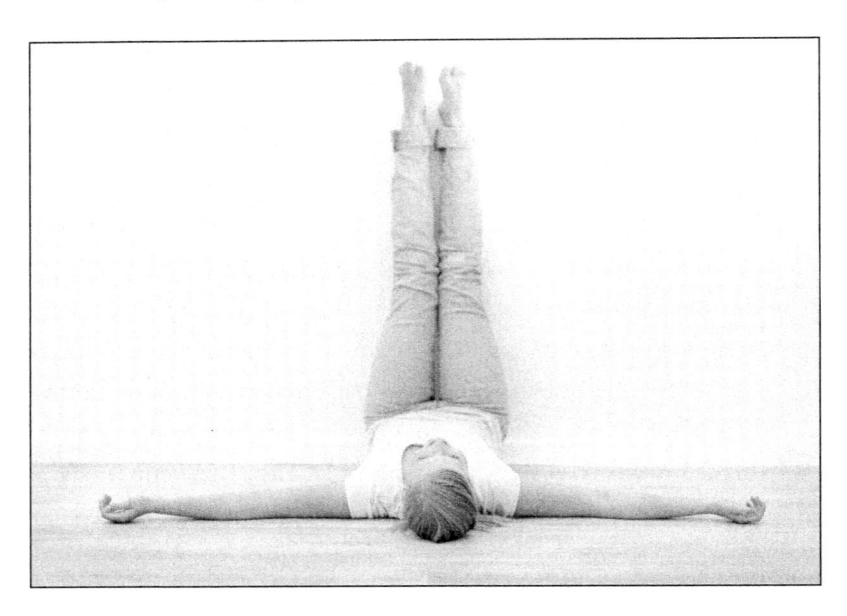

   Find a thick book or firm pillow and put a towel on top. Put both against a clear wall space. Sit beside the phone book, buttocks touching the wall, then reach out with the arm closest to the phone book, reach forward on the floor, so the chest comes close to the floor. Turn onto the book or pillow, so your buttocks are exactly in the middle on the book, and your legs are going up the wall. You must be fairly comfortable, close to the wall, so wiggle a bit until you find that comfort. Stay here inverted for five minutes or more. Let your arms be comfortably outstretched beside you on the floor. Your back is straight; your neck is long and your breathing is even and deep. Your feet will tingle or get a bit tired, but it is worth persevering for the longer stay. If it becomes too uncomfortable, don't force it but get used to it slowly over a period of weeks.

Always end your mini yoga session by relaxing in Savasana. It is that important.

Exercises for Cellulite Reduction

By now you realize that in order to diminish cellulite and reduce fat, it's important to get your body moving. The following exercises are targeted to the specific areas of your body that are prone to cellulite. Make sure to exercise; practice yoga or rebound at least once a day. And don't forget to hydrate!

Squats

Doing squats is great for toning the muscles in your thighs and buttocks. Stand with your feet apart a little wider than your shoulders, back straight and arms at a 90 degree angle in front of you. Inhale. Exhale, bending your knees slowly until you reach the classic squat position, as if you're going to sit down in a chair. For best results, hold for a few seconds, then inhale as you stand up. An easier way to get into the right form is to use a stability ball on your back against a wall, then squat leaning against it. Do ten squats then rest for a count of ten; repeat ten squats and work up to thirty squats. Don't forget to breathe. This will help with cellulite on your legs.

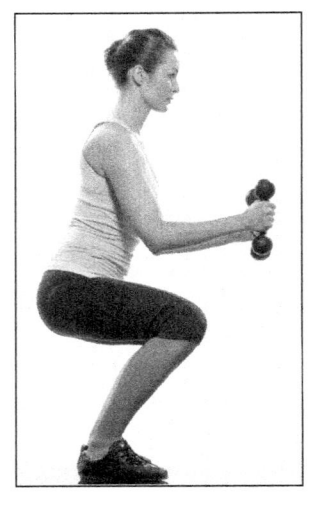

Buttock lift

Begin on all fours with a neutral spine on a yoga mat and place a blanket under your knees if you have sensitive knees.

Inhale as you raise your right leg until your thigh is even with your back, and then push your leg towards the ceiling. Exhale as you bring it back down to the original position. Do ten repetitions with the right leg, then ten with the left leg. Increase the repetitions to fifteen and then twenty as you progress. Don't forget to breathe. This exercise will give your buttocks a nice lift.

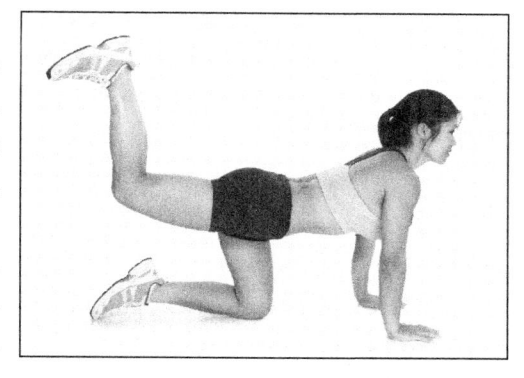

Raised buttock lifts

Lie on your back on your yoga mat, then place your feet on a sturdy chair that won't tip over. Place your palms on the floor with your arms at your sides. Inhale, and raise your thighs and buttocks towards the ceiling while contracting the back of your thighs and buttock muscles. Exhale as you lower your thighs and buttocks back down. Do ten repetitions, then fifteen and then twenty and hold the contraction for a few seconds each time.

Lunges

Stand straight with your right foot forward and left foot back about three feet apart. Hold light weights in each hand if desired. Exhale as you bend your knees to lower the body towards the floor. Keep your front knee behind your toes and be sure to lower straight down rather than forward.

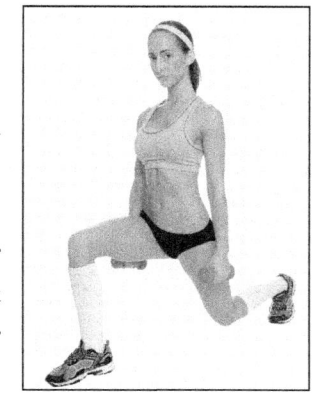

Keep your knee above your foot. Keep your torso straight and your abs in as you push through the front heel and back to starting position. Don't lock your knees at the top of the movement. Perform one to three sets of ten to fifteen repetitions, according to your fitness level and goals.

Inner thigh

Lie on your side on your yoga mat, using your arm with your elbow bent as a pillow for your head. Your other arm is in front of you with the palm on the mat as a brace to keep your upper body from falling forward. Align your legs with your body; inhale and exhale as you raise your leg up. You should feel this in the inner thigh. You can pulse while the leg is raised by moving your leg in small increments, focusing on your inner thigh, then, bring it back down. Do ten repetitions, then work up to twenty for one leg. Turn to the other side and do the same repetitions with the other leg.

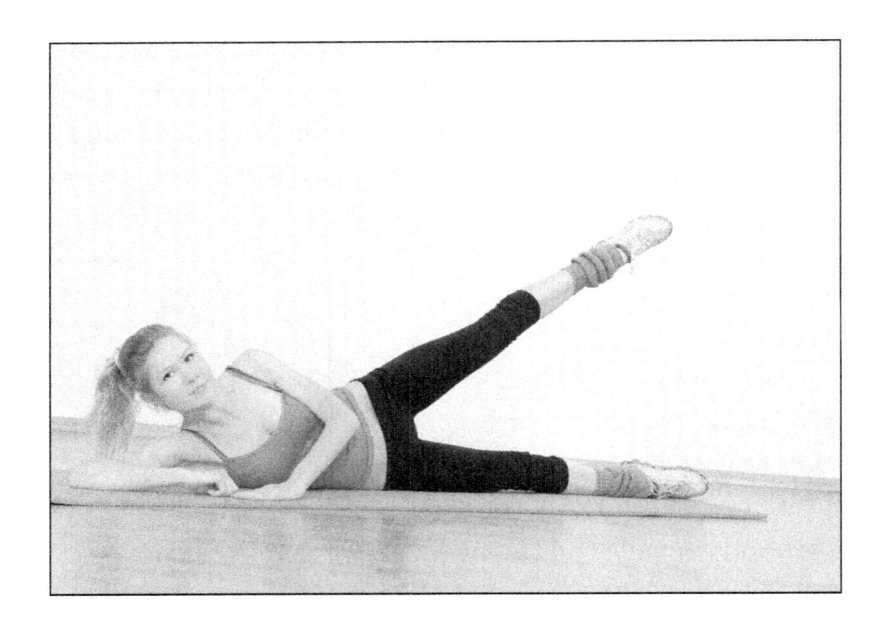

Burpees

You will need to wear running shoes for this exercise. Begin in a squat position with your hands on the floor in front; kick your feet back to a pushup position; immediately return your feet to the squat position then leap up as high as you can from the squat position. Repeat for a set of five and work up to ten; rest and then do another set. Burpees are an aerobic full body conditioning.

Stationary bodyweight lateral lunge/squat

Start by taking a wide stance with your feet and place your arms out straight in front of you. Shift your weight and hips to one side and squat down so your hips drop down behind that foot. Return to the starting position and repeat the same movement to the other side. Alternate this movement back and forth until the desired repetitions are met. Do a set of ten; rest and repeat. Don't forget to breathe!

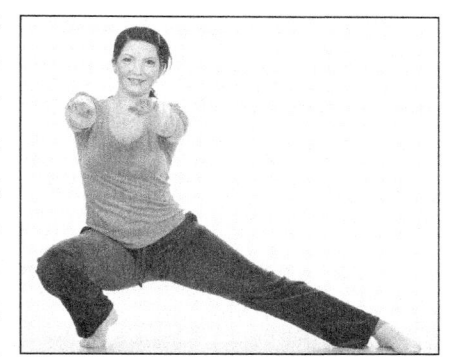

Bodyweight reverse lunge

Start by standing with your feet shoulder width apart. Step back with one foot and bend your knees into a lunged position. Your back knee should come close to touching the ground and your front leg should be bent to about 90 degrees at the knee. Maintain your upright posture throughout. Return to the starting position and repeat. Once repetitions are completed, repeat with the other leg. Do ten repetitions on each side; rest and do ten more. Work up to fifteen reps and then twenty.

Hip hikes

Start by lying face down on your yoga mat with your legs straight. Slowly raise one leg keeping it straight using just your gluteal muscles. Return to the starting position and do ten repetitions. Then repeat with the other leg.

Single leg kickbacks

Start in a four point position with your hands and knees on the yoga mat. Proceed to kick your leg back and up until you reach full extension. Squeeze your gluteal muscle while performing this movement. Then repeat with the other leg. For a more advanced movement you can attach an ankle weight around your leg. Do twenty reps on each side. Don't forget to breathe.

Bridging

Begin by lying on your back with your knees bent and feet on the yoga mat. Extend your arms out to steady yourself. Squeeze buttocks and raise your hips and lower back off the floor to form a straight line from your knees to your chest. Do not arch your back. Hold for five to ten seconds and slowly return to your starting position. Relax for five seconds. Repeat for ten reps and make sure to breathe!

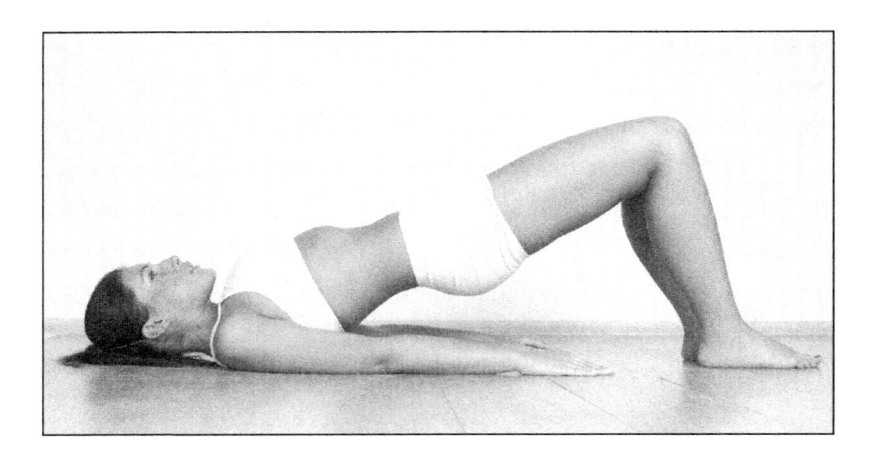

Side leg lifts
Start by kneeling on all fours on the yoga mat. Keeping your hips level, bring one leg out to the side. Think of the movement a dog does at a fire hydrant. Maintain your posture and balance and do not lean to the side while doing this exercise. Your back should stay flat. Do twenty reps on each side.

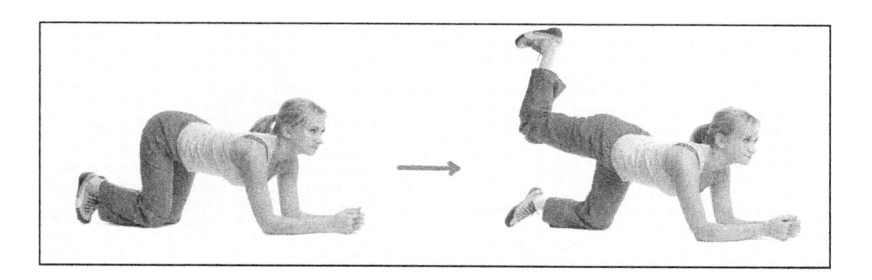

Tricep bench dip
This exercise will help with that nasty cellulite on the back of your arms! Start by placing your hands on the bench or sturdy chair. Your feet are on the floor with your legs semi straight. Proceed to bend your arms to about 90°. Return to the starting position; repeat for five reps and work up to ten.

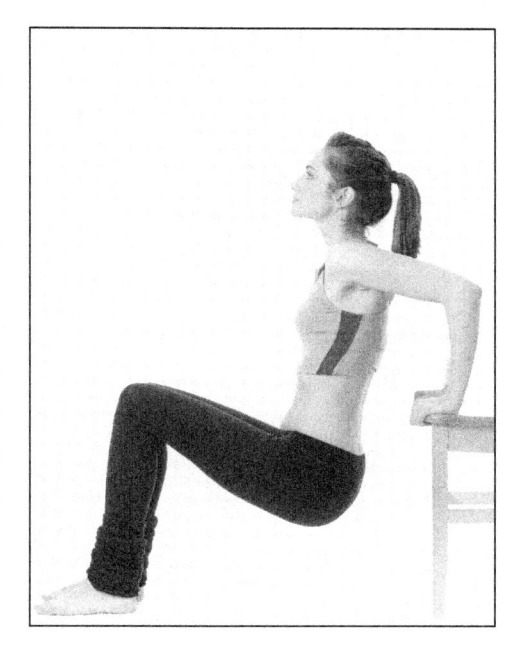

A SMOOTHER YOU

Band neutral grip curls

For this exercise, you will need bands which you can pick up at most fitness stores. Start by standing on the band with both feet and holding the handles. Keeping your grip neutral (palms facing down) curl the band up until your arms are at shoulder height, keeping your palms facing down. Return to the starting position and repeat for fifteen reps and then rest.

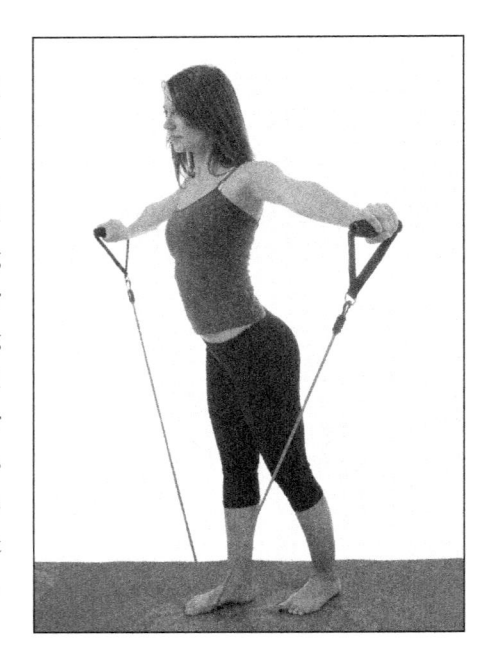

Bicep curl with band

Secure the band under your feet and hold the handles at waist level with your palms facing up. Curl your arms towards your shoulders with your palms facing up. Make sure to keep your elbows tucked in at your sides. Repeat for fifteen repetitions.

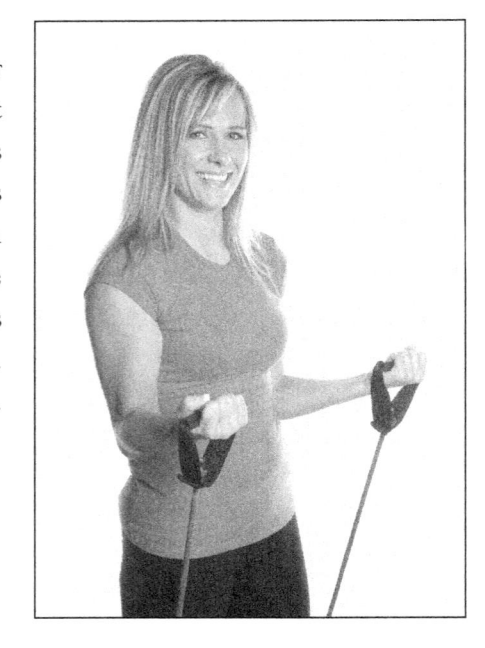

– 17 –

Meal Planning Guide for Cellulite Reduction

❖ **Each day**
- Before showering or bathing, exfoliate your buttocks, hips and thighs with a natural bristle dry skin brush.
- Once or twice a week, use an exfoliating scrub in the shower.
- Use our cellulite diminishing nutrient rich cream and massage it into your skin. (*Sold through Ara Wiseman Nutrition & Healing.*)
- Rebound for 15 minutes and/or do some Sun Salutations to get the lymph flowing.
- Prepare your food and water for the day.
- Make a conscious choice to eat healthy and stay positive and happy all day. Change your perception of the events currently happening in your life, by remembering that everything is happening for a reason. Be grateful for everything!
- Make sure to include 1 tablespoon ground chia seeds, flaxseeds or hemp seeds for the essential fatty acids, or take 2 flaxseed oil capsules.

❖ **Breakfast choices**
- Begin your day with hot or room temperature water with lemon.

- Green tea instead of coffee.
- Fresh vegetable juice, or fruit smoothie (*pages 134–136*).
- For a day of eating a lot of fruit have a smoothie with 4 bananas and 1 to 2 mangoes with enough water (1 liter/quart) to make it a creamy consistency. (You can also add 1 teaspoon barley grass powder or fresh cilantro). Remember that in preparation for consuming a lot of fruit, you must begin two or three days in advance by avoiding all fats from animal sources, over-consuming raw nuts and seeds, and using oils.
- Smoothie: 1 tablespoon sunflower lecithin (keep in refrigerator after opening); 1 scoop Sun Warrior brown rice protein powder; 1 tablespoon of wheat grass or barley grass powder; berries, banana and water or pure coconut water (no sugar added).
- Green shake with lots of fresh organic spinach or kale (*page 136*).
- High fiber gluten free cereal such as millet rice from Nature's Path with unsweetened almond milk and 1 tablespoon of ground flaxseed.
- Hot cereal such as millet, quinoa or buckwheat with blueberries and 1 tablespoon of ground flaxseeds or chia seeds. Add the ground seeds once the cereal is cooled to eating temperature.
- Two slices of Ezekiel 4.9 sprouted bread or gluten free bread with 1 tablespoon of almond butter and cinnamon or a few slices of an avocado.
- Buckwheat pancakes with fresh blueberries and cinnamon.
- Or you can have fresh fruit, eaten on its own, on an empty stomach until lunch or create fruit smoothies and have a full day of eating just fruit. (*Chapter 18, Recipes.*)

❖ Mid-morning snack choices
- Juice: carrot, apple, ginger or parsley (Juice Recipes, *pages 134–135*).

- Unsweetened coconut water (Vita Coco or Thirsty Buddha) with 1 tablespoon of greens.
- Fruit: berries, apple, banana, pear, orange, grapefruit or tangerine.
- Homemade energy bars (*page 162*).
- Raw veggie sticks with homemade low fat hummus, baba ganoush or cilantro pesto (*page 143*).
- High fiber muffin (*page 163*).
- Chia lemon drink: 1 liter of water, 1 tablespoon of chia, soak overnight in the fridge, in the morning add some fresh lemon or lime juice.
- Herbal tea such as licorice root, Essiac, Pau d'arco, mint, dandelion, rosehip, hibiscus or Tulsi.
- Half a cup of homemade guacamole with veggies or homemade flat bread crisps or buckwheat crackers (*page 162*).
- Unsweetened applesauce with a little cinnamon and 1 tsp of slippery elm (to help soothe the mucous membranes of the intestinal lining).
- A small handful of raw nuts or seeds. It is easier to digest one type of nut instead of a trail mix. Soak almonds overnight in pure filtered water to neutralize the enzyme inhibitors and unlock the valuable nutrients.
- A few organic unsulfured prunes, apricots, dates or figs.
- Steamed cabbage with red onion with light tamari.
- Steamed purple, white, and orange sweet potato with homemade cilantro pesto.

Make sure to drink plenty of water with greens such as wheat grass, barley grass or liquid chlorophyll throughout the day. Water naturally suppresses the appetite and flushes out toxins.

- ❖ Lunch choices
  - Liquid lunch. Juice: 3 broccoli florets, 1 garlic clove (if you're brave), 5 carrots, 2 tomatoes, 2 celery stalks and 1 red pepper. You can add cilantro and mint.
  - A cup of cooked lentil, mung bean, brown rice or quinoa pasta or buckwheat soba noodles with sautéed broccoli, cauliflower, zucchini, kale, mushrooms in low sodium veggie broth and topped with homemade pesto with pine nuts.
  - Peppers stuffed with buckwheat, millet or quinoa.
  - Millet patties with a large salad with lots of vegetables. Squeeze lemon juice on the salad or use our mango and tomato dressing, salsa or tahini dressing (*page 158*).
  - Lentil or chickpea salad with sprouted sunflower greens. You can add a few slices of avocado, use salsa, fresh lemon juice or a fruit dressing (*page 147*).
  - Ezekiel 4.9 whole grain wrap (found in the freezer section of the health food store) or a gluten free wrap with 1 tablespoon hummus, a few slices of avocado with grilled veggies, tomato, some tender green lettuce leaves and sprouts.
  - Grilled or poached wild salmon on salad greens.
  - Grilled veggies or the squash, chickpea and red lentil stew on salad greens with lemon juice (page 152).
  - Lentil, bean, squash and sweet potato, minestrone or green pea soup with half a cup of quinoa.
  - Cabbage salad with sliced avocado with two slices of gluten-free, Ezekiel 4.9 or Manna sprouted bread.
  - Cold asparagus soup or pepper and tomato soup (*page 138*) with a large salad with grated beets and carrots with fresh lemon juice or mango tomato dressing.
  - Quinoa salad with a lot of veggies and a ripe avocado with lemon juice dressing (*page 158*).

- Sprout salad: mung, lentil, adzuki, alfalfa, clover, sunflower and broccoli with sliced avocado, tomato slices and olives, dressed with mango tomato dressing or fresh lemon juice.
- Raw zucchini spaghetti with tomato sauce or homemade pesto.
- Cold mung bean pasta salad with tomato and avocado.

❖ **Mid-afternoon snack choices**
- Drink water with greens throughout the day.
- Apple slices.
- A small handful of raw soaked nuts and/or raw seeds with goji berries—only choose this if you haven't had any nuts yet (remember that it is easier on your digestion to have one kind of nut at a time as opposed to a trail mix).
- Green smoothie.
- Fruit smoothie.
- Celery, carrots, cucumber, peppers with homemade hummus or guacamole.
- A few Mary's wheat free crackers, rice crackers or any wheat free healthy crackers with 1 tablespoon of almond butter and 1 tablespoon of apple butter or cucumber slices with mustard.
- Vegetable juice made from any combination of the following or other vegetables of your choice: carrot, beet, celery, cabbage, bell peppers, dark leafy greens, a small amount of watercress or dandelion greens, parsley, cilantro, kale, ginger, sprouts, apple, and lemon.

❖ **Dinner choices**
- Begin with a salad of tender greens with vegetables of your choice, add some sunflower or broccoli sprouts with tahini, mango, tomato, or lemon dressing. You may add raw pumpkin or sunflower seeds, grated beets and carrots.

- An electrolyte broth: 3 cups pure water, chopped carrots, broccoli, dark leafy greens, celery, parsley, and 2 teaspoons miso paste.
- Vegetable soup with lots of vegetables, including potatoes, sweet potatoes, rutabaga, parsnips, broccoli, kale, cauliflower, squash, celery, peppers, carrots, zucchini, red cabbage—basically anything you have in your refrigerator. Begin with water, sautéed onions and fresh garlic, ginger, turmeric and curry; stir in low sodium vegetable stock and then add all the vegetables of your choice.
- A stir-fry with lots of different vegetables. Use 1/2 cup of organic coconut milk with curry powder or low sodium tamari sauce with fresh garlic, and sesame seeds.
- Squash and sweet potato soup over 1/2 cup of quinoa.
- Cooked lentils sautéed with onions and garlic, you can add spices or herbs, such as turmeric, curry, paprika, rosemary or tarragon. Add chopped veggies: tomatoes, celery, parsnips, carrots, potatoes, green beans, kale or collard greens. Decorate with chopped coriander if desired. To make into an Indian Dahl, add 2 tablespoons coconut milk and some curry spice and serve over Indian basmati rice or quinoa.
- Millet patties or sprouted mung bean patties with grilled or steamed veggies and a big salad.
- 1 cup of cooked lentil, chickpea, mung bean, quinoa or brown rice pasta with pesto, add sautéed vegetables.
- Mung bean or lentil patties with sautéed veggies and steamed sweet potato.
- Baked Falafel with steamed greens and a large salad (*page 151*).
- Artichoke Paella (*page 160*).
- As a side dish, steam broccoli, cauliflower, squash, sweet potato, carrots, bok choy, green beans, non GMO corn, and peas.

– 18 –

Recipes

The following section will help you prepare healthy food that is low in fat and tastes delicious. It starts with planning, so make sure to buy enough vegetables and the necessary ingredients needed to prepare food for the week. Low fat vegan living is a bit challenging in the beginning but if you stick to it, within about three weeks your taste buds will detect the sublime sweetness of red bell peppers, tomatoes, and even cabbage! Jicama root could become one of your favorites, as it is crispy, juicy, sweet, and excellent to munch on. Just peel and julienne one bulb and enjoy it for a healthy snack.

Some healthy guidelines to consider
- Buy organic, non GMO whenever possible. (*Refer to the Dirty Dozen/Clean 15 Charts on pages 171–172, for a list of fruits and veggies that are most contaminated with pesticides, and either avoid the Dirty Dozen or buy organic.*)
- Fresh vegetables and fruits are the best and frozen is next, dried is fine and canned is last.
- When altering a recipe remember, the fewer the ingredients, the more distinct the flavor and the easier it will be on your digestion. Foods that digest easily provide you with more energy, as opposed to making you feel tired after eating.
- Invest in a good juicer.

- Parchment paper is great for grilling vegetables or baking.
- In order to maintain a low fat healthy diet, try to limit using oils. Instead enjoy whole foods such as; avocados, olives, tahini, hummus, raw nuts and seeds, raw almond butter or homemade almond milk. Other foods to include are ground flaxseeds, chia or hemp seeds.
- Most of the recipes suggest to sauté with water, but you can also use low sodium vegetable stock, or a small amount of coconut oil (1 tablespoon) mixed with water if you prefer.
- To cut down on the fat in recipes, use zucchini or cauliflower to create the same texture you would get from nuts and seeds. For baking, use a ripe, mashed banana for a creamy texture and to replace fat. Bananas add nutrients like potassium, fiber, and vitamin B6. One cup of mashed banana works perfectly in place of a cup of butter or oil.
- In brownies and other dark baked goods, prune puree can replace butter or any fat. Prunes are high in antioxidants and contain nutrients such as vitamins A, K, boron and fiber. Combine 3/4 cup organic prunes with 1/4 cup boiling water, and puree to combine. Replace equal amounts of prune puree for butter in most dark baked good recipes.
- Chia seeds can be used in place of flour or cornstarch (which isn't healthy) to thicken sauces, gravies, burgers or even chocolate mousse and other desserts. It can also be used to replace eggs and fat in recipes.
- When it comes to salt, sea salt is a healthier choice than table salt, but keep in mind that it still contains the same amount of sodium (40%). Sea salt is obtained directly through the evaporation of seawater. It is usually unprocessed, or undergoes minimal processing, therefore retaining trace levels of minerals like magnesium, potassium, calcium and other nutrients.

- You can use a sodium substitute to decrease your overall sodium intake. Use lemon juice, lime juice, rosemary, basil, fresh garlic, pure garlic powder, cumin, nutmeg, cinnamon, fresh ground pepper, tarragon, thyme, oregano and other herbs and spices to add flavor to your meals. Celery replaces the salt in soup recipes. You can peel celery using a vegetable peeler to remove the strands.
- For soy sauce, switch to a lower sodium version or a light tamari, which is also gluten free! Unfortunately, even the lighter sodium alternatives still contain a considerable amount of sodium. To substitute a 1/2 cup of soy sauce in a recipe, mix 2 tablespoons light tamari with 3 tablespoons of water and 3 tablespoons fresh lime juice.
- Use tahini (sesame seed paste) instead of mayonnaise in dips and salad dressings. Tahini also makes a great dressing for vegetables. Not only are sesame seeds a very good source of manganese and copper, but they are also a good source of calcium, magnesium, iron, phosphorus, vitamin B1, zinc and fiber.
- Using applesauce in place of sugar can give a recipe the necessary sweetness without the extra calories. You can replace sugar for applesauce in a 1:1 ratio, but for every cup of applesauce you use, reduce the amount of liquid in the recipe by 1/4 cup.
- Another way to cut the sugar quantity in a recipe by half is by using pure vanilla extract. Next time you are baking cookies, try replacing 2 tablespoons of sugar with 1/2 tsp of vanilla bean powder.

HEALTHY JUICES

Potassium Juice

This is amazing for cleansing, neutralizing acids, rebuilding and reducing water retention (edema).

JUICE:

3 carrots

3 celery stalks

1/2 bunch spinach and parsley

Varicose Vein Tonic*

JUICE:

3 handfuls of dark greens made up of kale leaves, parsley, spinach, and watercress

5 carrots with green tops

1 green bell pepper

2 tomatoes

Skin Cleanser

JUICE:

1 cucumber with peel on

1/2 bunch fresh parsley

1 bunch alfalfa sprouts

3 – 4 sprigs of fresh mint

The Best Green Juice

JUICE:

1 cucumber

4 celery ribs

5 parsley sprigs

4 kale leaves

1/4 bulb fennel

5 asparagus spears
1 green apple
1/4 inch slice of ginger

VARIATION:
- You may also add a carrot or 1/4 beet.
- For anti-flu juice, add 1 large clove of garlic to the green juice but no carrot or beet.

Everything in the Fridge Must Go Juice
- Add many interesting greens to the juice including sprouts, beet greens, dandelion, kale, collard leaves and cilantro. Once you add these extra greens, add more cucumber to balance the taste.

Green Milk
JUICE:
5 celery ribs
1 long cucumber
2 handfuls of spinach or 3 kale leaves

IN THE BLENDER, BLEND:
1 cup almonds (soaked overnight in clean water then rinsed)
1 cup water
3 – 4 pitted dates
- Pour blended almond mush through a nylon mesh (also known as a nut milk bag) into a jug. Add the green juice and enjoy! This green milk has lots of protein and chlorophyll. It is so mild, even babies will happily drink it.

GREEN SHAKES

Green Shake with Berries
Fill your blender 3/4 full of baby kale or spinach
1 cup frozen or fresh berries of your choice
1 banana
1/2 – 1 cup pure filtered water or coconut water to blend to consistency of your choice.
- Add a few ice cubes if desired. Blend all ingredients together.

Green Shake with Apple and Banana
3 sprigs of watercress
1 green apple
1 lime
1/4 cucumber
4 mint leaves
1 banana
1/2 – 1 cup pure filtered water or coconut water to blend to consistency of your choice.
- Add a few ice cubes if desired. Blend all ingredients together.

Green Shake with Cucumber and Avocado
1 large English cucumber
1/2 lemon or lime, juiced
2 pitted dates to sweeten
1 small tomato
1/2 large avocado
2 handfuls of baby spinach leaves
Water or ice to fill the blender to 3/4 capacity.
- Blend until all ingredients are pureed. You may substitute any greens for the spinach, or 1/2 cup of soaked chia seeds for the avocado.

SOUPS

Basic Staple Cold Soup
- 1 medium ripe tomato
- 1 medium ripe avocado
- 1/2 English cucumber
- 1 small garlic clove
- A very small pinch of Celtic Sea salt or Himalayan pink salt
- 4-6 sprigs of cilantro
- 2 large handfuls of baby spinach or kale

- Slowly blend all ingredients with one cup of water. Add more water gradually for desired consistency—thinner for drinking or thicker for serving in a bowl. If serving in a bowl, sprinkle some hemp seeds on top for visual appeal, taste and of course high nutrition.

VARIATIONS:

To the above soup add or replace:
Add 3 stalks of celery chopped instead of sea salt
Add 1/4 small red onion instead of, or in addition to garlic
Add 1 tbsp coconut flakes instead of garlic
Add a thin sliver of ginger in addition to garlic
Add 1/2 red bell pepper instead of tomato
Add parsley instead of cilantro

- Replace spinach with romaine lettuce, mache (a gentle green), baby bok choy or kale. As you can see the choice is vast and fun to experiment with. Keep it simple and fast. These soups can be great for any meal or any time of the day—except late at night, when you should be sleeping and fasting.

Pepper and Tomato Soup

1 bell pepper, chopped

1 cup tomato, chopped

1/4 cup sundried tomatoes, soaked for 30 minutes

1 tbsp hemp seeds

1 tbsp red onion

1/2 garlic clove

3 stalks of celery chopped

1 handful fresh basil leaves

1 tbsp black olives, rinsed and chopped

1/4 cup of fresh cilantro chopped

- Blend the all the ingredients except olives until smooth. Pulse in basil and adjust seasoning. Decorate with olives and cilantro.

Asparagus Soup

1/2 cup water

1 cup carrots, diced

1 cup asparagus

1 tbsp raw tahini

1 clove garlic

1/2 tsp of Mrs. Dash

3 stalks of celery chopped

Lemon juice (optional)

- Start by blending the carrots, water, tahini, garlic, celery, lemon juice and Mrs. Dash until smooth, and then slowly add the asparagus. Blend everything and serve. Add seasonings to taste.

Potassium Soup

3 – 4 carrots, chopped
3 celery stalks, chopped
1/2 bunch parsley
2 potatoes with skins, scrubbed and cubed
1/2 head of cabbage, sliced (I prefer red cabbage)
1 onion, chopped
1 bunch of broccoli, sliced

- Sauté onions in a little coconut oil or use low sodium vegetable stock. You may add sliced garlic, ginger, turmeric and curry powder. Cook for a few minutes. Add all the vegetables then cover with filtered water or vegetable stock. Simmer for 30 minutes. Enjoy!

Sweet Potato and Squash Soup

1 medium onion, chopped
1 small piece of ginger, chopped
1 medium garlic clove, chopped
1 tsp turmeric (anti-inflammatory)
1 liter of low sodium vegetable stock
1 orange bell squash, peeled and cut into chunks
4 sweet potatoes, peeled and cut into chunks

- Sauté onions in veggie stock. Add ginger, garlic and turmeric. Sauté until onions are translucent. Add vegetable stock and a little water, chopped squash, celery and sweet potato. Cover and simmer for 30 minutes or until vegetables are soft. Puree the soup with a hand blender. You may add fresh nutmeg or cinnamon and serve over quinoa.

Minestrone Soup

- 1 large onion
- 4 large carrots
- 6 cups low sodium vegetable broth
- 3 zucchini
- 4 stalks celery
- 2 tbsp fresh basil, chopped
- 1 tbsp fresh oregano, chopped
  (if you can't find fresh, use dried)
- 1 tbsp fresh rosemary, chopped
- Pinch of sea salt
- 1/2 tsp black pepper
- 1 cup baby tomatoes (cut half of them into halves)
- 4 cloves garlic, minced
- 2 cups lentil or brown rice pasta, uncooked
- 2 cups cooked cannellini or navy beans,
  (can use canned and rinsed)

Dice the onion and cut the carrots into matchsticks. In a large saucepan, cook over medium heat for 3–5 minutes. If needed to keep the vegetables from sticking, add a small amount of water or broth. While waiting, cut the zucchini into matchsticks and slice the celery. Cook the pasta in a separate pot until its still a little undercooked. Add all remaining ingredients, except for the beans and pasta to the saucepan. Cover and bring to a simmer. Then add the pasta and reduce heat to medium low and cook for 10 minutes until pasta is tender. Remove the lid and stir in the beans until warmed.

Split Pea Soup

- 6 cups low sodium vegetable broth
- 1 cup filtered water
- 2 cups dried green split peas, rinsed
- 1 medium onion, chopped
- 1 cup carrots, chopped
- 4 potatoes peeled and chopped
- 3 celery ribs with leaves, chopped
- 2 garlic cloves, minced
- 1/2 tsp dried marjoram
- 1/2 tsp dried basil
- 1/4 tsp ground cumin
- Pinch of sea salt
- 1/4 tsp pepper
- 1/2 cup carrots, shredded
- 2 green onions, chopped

- In a large saucepan, combine all the ingredients except the shredded carrots and green onions and bring to a boil. Reduce heat, cover and simmer for 1 hour or until peas are tender, stirring occasionally. You may need to add more water. Cool slightly. Use a hand blender and puree the soup. Heat for 5 minutes. Garnish with shredded carrots and green onions.

Warming Winter Vegetable Soup

- 2 liters low sodium vegetable broth (I use two cartons of Pacific organic low sodium, or you can make your own)
- 1 large onion, diced
- 6 cloves of garlic, minced
- 2 bay leaves
- 1 tbsp fresh dill
- 2 carrots, sliced
- 2 stalks of celery, sliced

1 medium sweet potato, diced small
1 cup white mushrooms, sliced
2 cups broccoli
2 cups sliced green cabbage
1 handful of parsley, chopped
Sea salt and fresh pepper to taste

- Add 1 cup vegetable broth to a large soup pot and turn onto medium heat. Add bay leaves, dill, onions and sweet potatoes and sauté for 5 minutes. Add more broth if necessary to potatoes until they are almost covered.
- Add the mushrooms, garlic, carrots, celery, cabbage and the rest of one carton of vegetable broth. Stir and let it keep cooking over medium high heat for about 10 – 15 minutes. Add more vegetable broth if needed from the other carton. You want your vegetables to be almost done before adding the broccoli. Check on the sweet potatoes and if they are still too hard, keep cooking them until they are almost done. Add the remaining vegetable broth and bring it up to a boil. When it's boiling, turn it back down to medium high and add the broccoli and parsley. Cook for 2 – 4 minutes (depending on the size you cut them) and test the broccoli to make sure it's softer. Add sea salt and pepper and season to taste. Serve immediately.

DELICIOUS DRESSINGS AND DIPS

Cilantro Pesto*

    1-1/2 cups packed, fresh cilantro (stems and leaves about 1 bunch)

    2 cloves garlic

    3 tbsp fresh lemon juice

    1/4 – 1/2 cup of either pine nuts, sunflower or pumpkin seeds

    2 large peeled zucchini

- Combine all ingredients in food processor and process until the desired consistency or coarse paste is reached. This pesto can be stored in the fridge for up to a week. Put it on brown rice pasta, use it on sandwiches as a spread, or dip veggies into it. To make Basil pesto, replace the coriander with fresh basil and use pine nuts.

Delicious Hummus

    1 can of Eden brand chickpeas, drained and rinsed

    1 medium clove of garlic

    1 large heaping tbsp of tahini (I like the Artisana brand)

    2 tbsp fresh lemon juice

    Pinch of sea salt

    1/4 cup filtered water

- Put all ingredients into the food processor or blender and blend until smooth. Add the water slowly, to get the desired consistency. Can be stored in an airtight glass container in the fridge for a week.

Fruit Salsa

1 papaya chopped

3 mangos chopped

1 container of strawberries chopped

1 red onion chopped

A large handful of chopped fresh cilantro

1/4 cup of fresh mint chopped

2 limes, juiced

- Combine all the ingredients in a large bowl and mix, then serve and enjoy!

Salsa

1 jicama, peeled and diced

1 red bell pepper, finely chopped

1 yellow bell pepper, finely chopped

1 small red onion, finely chopped

1 Tbsp fresh mint leaves, minced

1 Tbsp fresh cilantro or basil leaves minced

1 lime, juiced

1/2 tsp minced garlic (optional)

- Mix all ingredients, and place in the fridge overnight.

Salsa Salad Dressing

2 ripe tomatoes, diced

1/2 cup green onions, minced

1 tsp ginger, minced

1 tsp fresh mint, minced

1 tsp lime juice

Sea salt and pepper to taste

- Mix all ingredients and place in the fridge overnight.

Dressing for Steamed Veggies or Salads

1 tbsp tahini (sesame seeds ground into butter)

Juice of 1 lemon or lime

Pinch of Celtic sea salt or Himalayan pink salt

- Stir all the ingredients together and add some water if needed.

Spicy Flax Dressing

1 tbsp fresh lemon juice

1 tbsp chopped chives

1 tbsp chopped parsley

1/2 tsp fresh basil

1/2 tsp oregano

1/2 tsp mustard

1 small clove garlic, roughly chopped

3 tbsp flaxseed oil

Pinch of cayenne

Pinch of sea salt

- Blend everything except the oil in the food processor, then add the 3 tbsp of oil in through the top part of the processor until creamy. Place the above ingredients into a dark glass container and use immediately. To store, seal tightly in a small dark container and refrigerate. (*Please note that flax seed and hemp seed oil are heat, light and oxygen sensitive. When using these oils, measure a small amount sufficient for only one or two uses. Otherwise, rancidity will nullify all the benefits.)

Creamy Dressing for Steamed Veggies

1/2 a medium ripe avocado

Juice of 1 lemon

1 Ataulfo (yellow honey) mango

4–6 sprigs of cilantro

Pinch of a sea salt
- Blend well to make a creamy dressing. You may add other spices to further liven up the taste buds, such as fresh or dried basil, oregano, tarragon, mustard, curry, cumin or coriander powder.

Great Salad Dressing

1 cup freshly squeezed orange juice
2 medjool dates, pitted
1 tbsp fresh lemon juice
1 tbsp fresh ginger, minced
1/3 cup raw unsalted cashews (soaked for a few hours in cold filtered water)
1/4 cup chopped peeled zucchini (or half a zucchini)
Pinch of sea salt and fresh pepper
- Place all the ingredients in the food processor and process until smooth. Best used within 3 days (due to fresh orange juice which is perishable).

Ceasar Salad Dressing

1/3 cup water
3 tbsp fresh lemon juice
1 tbsp Dijon mustard
1 tbsp tahini
1/4 cup chopped peeled zucchini
1 tbsp Nama Shoyu or low sodium Tamari sauce
2 cloves of garlic chopped
- Blend all ingredients in food processor or blender until smooth. May be refrigerated in a glass jar for a week.

Creamy Thai Dressing

1 large ripe avocado
3/4 of a large tomato
Small slice of red onion
Small slice of jalapeño pepper
1 small lime, juiced
1 – 2 small handfuls of cilantro
Small piece of fresh ginger

- Blend all the ingredients together in a blender or food processor.

Strawberry Dressing

1 cup strawberries
1/2 orange juiced
1/2 tbsp freshly grated ginger
1 tbsp sprouted chia powder
3 dates pitted
1/4 cup water

- Blend all the ingredients in a food processor. Place in a glass container and store overnight in the fridge to allow the dressing to thicken.

SALADS AND OTHER RECIPES

A Kale Salad Even Kids Love!

4 – 6 large leaves of kale, stems removed
1 tbsp of coconut oil
1 large cloves of garlic
Juice of 1 large lemon
1 tsp of sea or Himalayan salt

- Slice kale leaves into long strips and place in a large bowl.
- Slowly sprinkle sea salt on kale leaves. Massage gently with your hands for about five minutes until leaves are wilted. Add oil, keep massaging. Add chopped garlic and lemon. Set the bowl aside to rest for an hour. This will break down the cellulose of the kale leaves making them easier to digest and allowing the flavor to deepen. To serve, you may top with chopped tomatoes, sliced avocados and/or hemp seed nuts.

Kale Salad Dressing

2/3 cup sliced strawberries, raspberries or tomatoes
1/4 cup balsamic vinegar
1/2 shallot, chopped
2 tsp fresh thyme leaves
1-1/4 tsp Dijon mustard
1/4 tsp ground black pepper
1/4 cup filtered water

- Blend together in with 1/4 cup water in a blender and blend until very smooth.

Cabbage Salad

1/2 shredded (chopped) red cabbage
1 cup thinly sliced green beans
1 clove garlic, minced

Sea salt and pepper to taste
Fresh lemon juice
1/4 cup sesame seeds

- Combine all the ingredients and serve.

Lentil Salad

2 cups lentils (canned is fine, rinsed)
2 oranges, sectioned (without skin or seeds)
1 red onion, thinly sliced
2 cloves garlic
4 tbsp chopped fresh parsley
1/4 of a chopped hot pepper
Juice of 1 lemon
1/2 cup chopped fresh cilantro
Sea salt and pepper to taste

- Mix all ingredients and serve.

Spinach Salad

4 cups organic baby spinach
2 ribs of celery, finely sliced
1/2 cup of peeled, chopped cucumber
2 scallions, finely chopped
1/2 cup of grape tomatoes chopped

DRESSING INGREDIENTS:

1 small avocado
1 medium tomato
1/2 lime juice

- Place all the salad ingredients into a bowl. Blend the avocado, tomato and lime juice in a blender and pour over the salad.

Avocado Salad

1 English cucumber finely chopped

1 large ripe avocado (diced)

1/2 red onion (sliced thin)

1 tbsp fresh cilantro (minced)

Pinch of sea salt

2 tbsp fresh lime juice

1 tsp ground pepper (fresh)

- In a large bowl, combine all ingredients and mix thoroughly. Chill until ready to serve.

Pasta Salad

3 cups lentil, quinoa or brown rice pasta

3 ripe tomatoes, chopped

1 large ripe avocado chopped

1 small clove of garlic crushed or minced

1/2 cup chopped fresh cilantro

2 tbsp fresh lime juice

Pinch of sea salt

Freshly ground pepper to taste

- Cook the pasta until it is al dente. Drain and rinse under cold water until pasta is cooled. Combine all the rest of the ingredients in large bowl and add the pasta and mix. Chill until ready to serve.

Sweet Potato Vegetable Stew

1/2 of a squash peeled, seeded and chopped

2 sweet potatoes peeled and sliced

3 or 4 white potatoes peeled and sliced

A few cauliflower and broccoli florets

1 red bell pepper chopped

■ Put into a pot and add half of a container of low sodium veggie stock and cook on medium heat for 5 minutes, then reduce heat, and cover and cook for 20 minutes, stirring occasionally and adding a little more veggie stock if necessary.

Honey Roasted Root Vegetable Medley

1 carrot, peeled, in 3/4 inch slices
1/2 sweet potato (about 4 oz.), peeled in 1-inch cubes
1 turnip, peeled in 1-inch cubes
1/2 parsnip, in 3/4 inch slices
1 yellow beet, peeled, in 1-inch cubes
2 garlic cloves, peeled and chopped
2 tbsp balsamic vinegar
1 tbsp unpasteurized raw honey
1 tbsp fresh rosemary, finely chopped
Pinch of sea salt
Fresh ground black pepper, to taste

■ Combine balsamic vinegar, honey, garlic, rosemary, salt and pepper in shallow glass dish. Add vegetables and toss so they are evenly coated. Cover the glass dish with foil or an ovenproof lid. Set oven to 350°F and roast for 30 minutes or until all vegetables are soft throughout. Toss vegetables and remove foil or lid and cook 5 more minutes.

Falafel

4 cups stemmed and torn collard greens or Swiss chard
1/2 cup fresh cilantro
2 cups canned chickpeas, rinsed and drained
2 cloves garlic
1-1/2 tbsp tahini
1-1/2 tbsp fresh lemon juice
1/2 tsp cumin

1/4 tsp turmeric
1/4 tsp Sea salt
1/4 tsp black pepper
3-4 tbsp spelt flour

- Add everything except spelt flour to a food processor and process until mixture is smooth. You may need to scrap down the sides and process again for a minute or two. Then transfer to a bowl and add the flour 1 tbsp at a time until the mixture is thick enough to make into balls. Place the balls on a cookie sheet lined with parchment paper. Set oven to 350°F and bake for 10 minutes, turn them over and bake another 5-10 minutes. They should be crispy on the outside and soft on the inside. Dip into tahini dressing and enjoy!

Squash, Chickpea and Red Lentil Stew

1 can (540 ml) no salt added chickpeas, drained and rinsed
1/2 large butternut squash (about 1-1/2 lbs.), peeled, seeded and cut into 1-inch cubes
4 large carrots, peeled and cut into 1/2 inch pieces
1/2 sweet onion, chopped
1/2 cup dry, red lentils
4 cups low sodium vegetable broth
2 tbsp tomato paste
1 tbsp minced peeled fresh ginger
1 tbsp Mrs. Dash

- Add onion, squash and carrots to a stainless steel frying pan and lightly sauté using water or vegetable stock. Once onions are translucent transfer to an oven proof glass bowl and add the rest of the ingredients. Place in oven and bake at 350°F for 30 minutes, stirring occasionally. Serve over ½ cup of quinoa, brown or white Indian basmati rice.

Lentil Veggie Burgers

1 cup cooked lentils
2 cloves of garlic
1 small onion
1 tbsp raw unsalted sunflower seeds
1 tbsp raw unsalted pumpkin seeds
1 tbsp apple cider vinegar
1 tsp turmeric
1 tsp ground cumin
1 tsp chili powder
1/2 cup packed cilantro
1 tbsp chia seed powder (it will thicken the mixture by absorbing any liquid)
1 large chopped carrot

- Process the onion and garlic first in the food processor with the pulse, until the onion is finely chopped. Then add the remaining ingredients. You may need to turn it off and scrape down the sides and continue to process. Let it sit for 5 or so minutes to let the chia absorb and then form into patties. Place on baking sheet lined in parchment paper and bake at 350°F for 10 minutes. Then flip and cook for another 10 minutes to desired texture. You can place on an Ezekiel 4.9 sprouted wrap or a lettuce leaf with mustard and relish or try some horseradish for something different with cut up tomatoes and lettuce.

Thai Basil Curry

CURRY PASTE:

1 cup firmly packed basil leaves
1 medium shallot, coarsely chopped
1/4 cup firmly packed cilantro
1 tbsp fresh mint
1 tbsp Thai green chili paste

1 tbsp grated fresh ginger

2 garlic cloves, peeled

VEGETABLES:

1/2 eggplant, cut into 1-inch pieces

1 zucchini, cut into 1-inch pieces

1/2 red bell pepper, cut into 1-inch pieces

1/2 green bell pepper, cut into 1-inch pieces

1/4 cup coconut milk

1/4 cup low-sodium vegetable broth

2 tbsp water

2 tbsp lime juice

Sea salt and pepper to taste

- Place all the vegetables in an oven-proof glass bowl. You may want to line the bottom of the bowl with parchment paper so the vegetables don't stick. Bake at 350°F for 15 minutes, or until vegetables begin to soften. Meanwhile, make the curry paste: Place all ingredients in a blender or food processor, and pulse until a smooth paste forms, adding a little water if necessary. Stir curry paste, coconut milk and broth into the vegetables. Cover and cook for 15 minutes, or until vegetables are tender, stirring occasionally. Season with salt and pepper, and serve with jasmine rice.

Vegetable Kasha

2 carrots, sliced

1/4 cup canned chickpeas

1 onion, chopped

1 clove garlic, chopped

2 tsp Mrs. Dash

2-1/4 cups plum tomatoes, chopped

1 cup buckwheat (kasha)

1 cup mushrooms, sliced

1/2 a green pepper

1/2 a red pepper

Sea salt and pepper to taste

1 cup sunflower sprouts

- Sauté the onions and garlic in water until onions are translucent. Add tomatoes, vegetables and chickpeas and sauté until all the vegetables are soft. Meanwhile heat 2 cups of filtered water, stir in 1 cup of buckwheat and cook until water is dissolved and buckwheat is soft. Add sautéed vegetables to cooked buckwheat and stir. You can add some chopped fresh cilantro or basil. Add the sunflower sprouts on top.

Simple Grilled Vegetables

1 red pepper, sliced

1 zucchini, sliced

1 eggplant, sliced in 1/2 inch circles

10 small potatoes sliced

1 sweet potato peeled and sliced

1 tsp Mrs. Dash

1 handful of fresh rosemary chopped

1 clove garlic chopped

Fresh lemon juice optional

- Place vegetables on baking sheet on top of a large piece of parchment paper. Add rosemary, chopped garlic, Mrs. Dash and lemon juice and a little water and fold parchment paper with vegetables inside and seal by folding the paper a few times to create the seal. Cook vegetables at 375°F for 20 minutes. Open the sealed parchment paper carefully as the steam will escape and it is very hot. If the potatoes are still too hard cook for another 5 minutes with the paper opened.
- Serve on top of a salad or as a side dish with other meals or as a meal with tahini dressing.

Simple Steamed Vegetables

3 potatoes peeled and cut into larger pieces
1 large sweet potato peeled and cut into larger pieces
2 zucchinis cut into larger pieces
3 carrots peeled and chopped and cut into pieces
2 bunches of bok choy washed with separated leaves
1 head of broccoli cut into smaller pieces

- Place all the vegetables into a steamer. I use a stainless steel pot with a stainless steel steamer basket. Put enough water at the bottom of the pot. Cover and cook until vegetables are soft. Serve with tahini mustard dressing.

TAHINI MUSTARD DRESSING

1 tbsp tahini
A little water to get desired consistency
1 tsp mustard

- Stir together in bowl.

Coconut Cauliflower Stew*

1 tbsp coconut oil
2 medium onions chopped
2 large carrots chopped
2 large garlic cloves minced
1 tbsp grated fresh ginger
1-2 tbsp curry powder
1/4 tsp cayenne pepper
1 tsp sea salt
2 fist-sized orange sweet potatoes, diced
3 cups diced cauliflower
1 red bell pepper chopped
1/2 cup chickpeas drained and rinsed
1/2 can low fat coconut milk

1/4 – 1/2 cup filtered water or vegetable stock

1/4 shredded unsweetened coconut

1 handful chopped fresh cilantro

- Heat the oil or use low sodium vegetable stock in a soup pot on medium then add the onions and sauté for 5 minutes. Add the carrots, garlic, ginger, curry powder, cayenne and salt and sauté for 5 minutes. Stir in sweet potatoes, cauliflower, red pepper, chickpeas, coconut milk, water or vegetable stock and shredded coconut. Cover and cook for about 15 minutes, stirring occasionally until sweet potatoes are soft. Garnish with cilantro when serving.

Portabella Mushrooms with Salsa

4 portabella mushrooms cleaned and stalks removed

2 tsp lemon juice

1 tbsp low sodium tamari

Sea salt and pepper to taste

SALSA:

1 ripe tomato, diced

1/2 cup green onions, minced

1 tsp ginger, minced

2 tsp fresh mint, minced

1 tsp lime juice

Sea salt and pepper to taste

- Rub lemon juice, tamari, sea salt and pepper on portabella mushrooms. Bake on baking sheet lined with parchment paper at 350°F for 20 minutes. When the mushrooms are soft, they are cooked. Mix salsa ingredients together in a bowl, and spoon over baked mushrooms and serve.

Quinoa Salad

4 cups of water
2 cups quinoa
1 large English cucumber
4 celery stalks
1 red and 1 yellow pepper
2 tomatoes
A bunch of cilantro
1 soft avocado

- Add quinoa to water and bring to a boil then lower the heat, cover and simmer until all the water is absorbed. Remove from heat and uncover to let it cool. Meanwhile chop the rest of the ingredients into small pieces and place in a large bowl. Add the cooled quinoa and mix. You can add lemon juice and sea salt to taste or you can use one of the dressings in the salad dressing section. Serve and enjoy!

Millet Patties

1 cup dry millet
2 cups of boiling water
1/4 cup onions, finely chopped
1 tsp ground oregano or thyme
2 tsp coconut oil
1/4 cup seasoned organic corn meal or oatmeal for breading the patties
2 tbsp Nama Shoyu or low sodium Tamari
1/2 tsp garlic powder
1/2 cup fresh parsley, minced
1 tsp oregano or thyme
3 tbsp sesame seeds

- In a medium saucepan, add millet to boiling water, cover and cook for 45 minutes. Meanwhile, in a small frying pan sauté the onions and spices in the coconut oil until soft. (Add a little water if needed to prevent sticking). In another large bowl, thoroughly combine the cooked millet, sauteed onion mixture and remaining ingredients. Form into patties, and coat each patty with the seasoned cornmeal. Bake at 350°F on a baking sheet lined with parchment paper until browned, approximately 25 – 35 minutes. Flip once to brown on both sides, or you can sauté them gently first in coconut oil on a medium heat until brown.

Sprouted Mung Bean Patties*

1 cup sprouted mung beans (mung beans are easy to sprout)
1 cup cooked chick peas
2 – 3 heaping tbsp of raw sunflower and pumpkin seeds
1 egg (for vegans, replace with 1 tbsp ground flaxseeds mixed with 3 tbsp warm water)
1 big green chili or jalapeno (You can toss out the seeds to reduce the heat)
2 garlic cloves minced
2 tbsp apple cider vinegar
1 heaping tbsp of cumin powder
1 tsp ancho chili powder
Sea salt and pepper
1 small red onion chopped
Fistful of cilantro chopped
1 tbsp coconut oil

- Blend all ingredients in food processor and then form into patties. Heat 1 tbsp coconut oil on medium heat. Sauté the patties gently, two at a time. Reduce heat to medium-low and cover the pan with the lid and let each patty cook for a good 5 minutes on each side. Flip carefully when browned. The trick is to cook patties slowly all the way through on low heat.

Only then does their texture become chewy. Enjoy with a quinoa salad or as a sandwich topped with onion, lettuce, tomato and hummus.

Artichoke Paella*

- 1 cup brown rice
- 2 cups boiling water
- 2-1/2 cups vegetable broth
- 1 onion chopped
- 2 cloves of garlic, crushed or minced
- 3/4 cup julienned green bell pepper
- 3/4 cup julienned red bell pepper
- 1 can lima beans rinsed and drained or frozen baby lima beans, thawed
- 2 small tomatoes, chopped
- 1 tsp dried oregano
- Pinch of sea salt
- 1/8 tsp crushed red pepper flakes
- Pinch of saffron
- 1 can or glass container (15 oz) water-packed artichoke hearts drained and cut in halves
- 1 cup frozen peas, thawed

- Put the rice in a glass bowl and pour the boiling water over it. Cover and let stand for 20 minutes while you prepare the remaining ingredients. After 20 minutes, drain off extra water and set the rice aside. Heat the vegetable broth to boiling in a saucepan. Scoop out 1/3 cup of the broth into a wok or large skillet with sloping sides. Add the onion and garlic and stir over medium heat until the onion softens about 3 minutes. Add the green and red peppers, lima beans, and tomatoes and cook, stirring about 3 minutes. Stir in the oregano, sea salt, pepper flakes, saffron and the reserved rice and the remaining hot broth. Bring to boil, reduce the heat, cover and cook for 30 minutes. Stir in the artichokes and peas. Remove the pan from the heat, cover, and let stand 5 minutes before serving.

Vegan Black Bean Chili

    1 large sweet onion, diced
    1 large carrot, diced
    5 white mushrooms, diced
    8 cloves of garlic, minced
    1 red bell pepper, diced
    29 oz. can black beans, drained (Eden Organic)
    28 oz. can crushed tomatoes (Eden Organic)
    1 tsp cumin
    1 tsp paprika
    1/2 tsp chili powder
    1 tsp honey
    Low sodium vegetable stock
    1 tsp Mrs. Dash
    Sea salt and pepper to taste

- In a large pot, sauté onions, mushrooms and carrots for approx. 7 minutes on medium heat in a small amount of low sodium vegetable stock. Add the garlic and red pepper and sauté for 5 more minutes, stirring occasionally. Add water if necessary to keep from burning. Add the tomatoes and drained beans and seasonings and heat through for about 15 minutes, until carrots are soft. Serve with brown rice or baked sweet potatoes.

Raw Zucchini Pasta with Raw Tomato Sauce

    2 medium-sized zucchini, spiralized
    3 organic tomatoes (quartered)
    4 to 5 sun dried tomatoes (soaked)
    2 garlic cloves (chopped)

1 shallot (chopped)

5 fresh basil leaves

- Spiralize zucchini into noodles and set aside (you can purchase a Saladacco Spiral Slicer to make vegetable pasta). Add all ingredients for sauce into a food processor and blend until smooth. You may need to add a little water to get desired consistency.

Flat Bread Crisps

4 large Ezekiel 4.9 wraps (found in the freezer section of the health food store)

1 tbsp of melted coconut oil

1 tbsp chopped fresh basil leaves or rosemary

Pinch of sea salt

- Preheat oven to 375°F. Cut wrap into triangles. Line baking sheet with parchment paper. Place triangles in a single layer on the parchment and lightly brush with coconut oil and sprinkle evenly with basil or rosemary and sea salt. Bake in preheated oven for 8 to 12 minutes or until light brown and crisp.

Energy Bars*

1-1/2 cups pitted prunes and dates

1/3 cup organic unsweetened cocoa powder

1/3 cup chia seeds

3/4 tsp vanilla extract

1 cup raw walnut pieces (walnuts are high in essential fatty acids)

Coconut or almond flour for dusting

- Place dates and prunes in a food processor and puree until thick paste forms. If the mixture seems dry, you can slowly add small amounts of warm water, just enough to moisten. Add cocoa powder, chia seeds, vanilla and combine. Then add walnuts and pulse until nuts are finely chopped and well distributed. Spread large sheet of waxed paper on work surface and dust with coconut or almond flour. Transfer mixture to wax paper and press mixture into 1/2 inch thick rectangle. Wrap tightly with the waxed paper and then in foil and chill overnight. Unwrap block and cut into 10 bars. Dust edges with coconut or almond flour, then wrap each bar in waxed paper and store in refrigerator.

Blueberry Buckwheat Muffins

DRY INGREDIENTS:

1/4 cup buckwheat flour

3/4 cup + 4 tbsp spelt flour

1/2 tsp non-aluminum baking powder

1/4 tsp baking soda

1/2 tsp cinnamon

1/4 cup coconut sugar

WET INGREDIENTS:

1/2 cup unsweetened applesauce

1/4 cup almond milk

1 tbsp ground flaxseeds mixed with 3 tbsp water

1 tbsp melted coconut oil

1 tsp vanilla extract

1/2 tsp almond extract

1/2 cup frozen blueberries, thawed

Muffin cup cake liners

- Preheat oven to 375°F. Place cupcake liners in muffin tins. Combine dry ingredients in a medium bowl. Combine all wet ingredients, then add to dry ingredients. Mix until just combined and then fold in blueberries. Pour into muffin tins. Bake for 16 – 18 minutes. Check with a toothpick after 15 minutes.

DESSERTS

Banana Ice Cream

4 bananas peeled (frozen)
1 tbsp milled chia
1 tbsp dark organic cacao
1/4 tsp pure vanilla extract
1/4 tsp cinnamon
1/4 tsp ground cardamom (optional)

- Place all ingredients together in a food processor and allow the motor to run until it's smooth and creamy. Stop and break up large clumps with a spatula as needed.

Raw Blueberry Pie*

CRUST:

1-1/2 cup packed pitted raw dates
1 oz coconut flakes
1 oz raw almonds

- Put the raw almonds and coconut in the food processor and pulse twice, add the dates next and process until it becomes a large ball. Squish this mixture on the pie pan until it's even and flat.

FILLING:

1 cup packed soft pitted raw dates
3-1/2 cups blueberries (2 cups for the filling, 1 cup FRESH blueberries to mix into the filling, 1/2 cup to top)

- *In the food processor*:
Bend 2 cups of the blueberries with 1 cup of dates until it becomes a smooth paste. Then fold in the fresh blueberries. Pour the mixture into the pie pan and top with the leftover blueberries. Place into the freezer for 30 minutes and then devour your low fat raw vegan blueberry pie recipe!

Apple Crumble

FRUIT BOTTOM:

5 medium to large apples, cored and sliced (I like to keep the peel on)

2 tbsp spelt flour (for gluten free use brown rice or almond flour)

1 tbsp cinnamon

1 tbsp Sucanat or coconut sugar

- Toss sliced apples in flour, cinnamon and coconut sugar.

Spread the mixture on the bottom of a parchment lined oven proof glass bowl.

CRUMBLE TOPPING:

3 tbsp coconut oil

1 tbsp applesauce

1/2 cup of spelt flour or use gluten free option

2/3 cup of rolled oats

1/2 cup of Sucanat or coconut sugar

3 tsp of cinnamon

- In a separate bowl combine the coconut oil, applesauce with the oats, flour, sugar, and cinnamon and mix. Spread the crumble over the apples. Bake at 350°F for 30 minutes. Serve and enjoy!

Chocolate Coconut Macaroons

2 cups shredded coconut

3 tbsp coconut oil

6 tbsp cocoa powder

2 tbsp maple syrup

1/2 tsp pure vanilla

- Put shredded coconut into a food processor and pulse several times to make the coconut finer. Add remaining ingredients and process again until mixed. Form mixture into round balls and place on parchment paper and refrigerate for 15 minutes or until firm. Enjoy!

TEAS

Enzyme Digestive Tea ❙ Steep 2 parts peppermint and hibiscus and 1 part papaya leaf and rosemary in boiling water for ten minutes in a covered glass or ceramic pot with mesh screen. Or simmer in a pot and then strain.

Pau D'arco Tea is another favorite. It can be purchased from health food stores as loose tea or in bags and has a multitude of benefits. It has been used to get rid of fungus or yeast in the system, for skin problems, varicose veins, psoriasis and the list goes on.

Rooibos Tea does not have caffeine and is delicious as a chai base. You can steep the tea either loose or in bags, and add cinnamon sticks, sliced ginger root chopped, sliced turmeric root, star anise, cloves, cardamom powder or the pods, peppercorns and fennel seeds. To sweeten use raw honey or a little coconut sugar, and add some almond milk if you wish.

Dandelion Tea is good for your liver and contains potassium, which is helpful for any edema (swelling) or water retention.

Essiac Herbal Tea* helps to remove excess fatty deposits in artery walls, heart, kidney and liver. It removes some of the toxic accumulations in the fat and helps to neutralize acids, absorbs toxins in the bowel, and eliminates both. (**Do not use if pregnant or breastfeeding. Always start out with a small amount.*)

– 19 –

Tidbits to Chew On

- Digestion begins in your mouth. Chew your food thoroughly to mix the food with the enzymes in your saliva, for easier and more complete digestion.

- It takes 20 minutes for your digestive system to communicate satiety to your brain. If you eat quickly or while watching television or reading, you will end up eating too much.

- Health is wealth. Make sure your priorities are set straight. How much money you are willing to spend on your car versus your food—is a good indicator of your priorities.

- Pause every time you are about to eat and ask, "Am I nourishing myself with this food I'm about to eat?" It will help you become more mindful of your choices.

- Know the meaning of *junk food*. It is not food; it is pure junk dressed up in a seductive manner to look like food.

- Chemicals, sodium, fat, and sugar are added to fast, convenience foods to bypass your brain's satiety mechanism, making you eat more and crave it. Your taste buds eventually become numb to the taste of real, unprocessed whole foods that contain naturally occurring sodium and fat, along with all the vitamins, fiber, water, and minerals needed to metabolize it efficiently.

- Refined simple carbohydrates are sugars found in packaged cookies, cakes, soda etc. They have a negative effect on your blood sugar levels and mood, are acid forming and should not be consumed.

- Most people snack because they have not met their caloric and nutritional needs. Once you start consuming the right amount of healthier nutrient dense foods, you will reduce your need for continuous snacking.

- When setting a goal, it's important to be realistic about what your body is capable of achieving, at whatever stage of life you are in.

- Learn to slow down, and don't eat when you are stressed. When you are under stress you are not producing adequate digestive enzymes, and you are unable to digest properly.

- Drinking fluids with your meal dilutes your digestive juices, which impairs your digestion. Limit the amount of liquid you consume with your meals to approximately four ounces or less of room temperature fluid. Drink pure, filtered water between meals.

- Follow proper food combining (avoid mixing fat with starch and eat fruit alone). Simplify your food combinations.

- Do not eat a heavy meal late at night—aim for at least three hours without food before you lie down for bed.

- Ensure a minimum of 25 grams of fiber, 5–10 servings of fruits and vegetables (raw and lightly steamed vegetables for enzymes, vitamins and minerals) every day.

- Start to pay attention to sodium, sugar, and unhealthy fats in food. Don't be fooled by the smiling faces on the box.

- Maintain a food diary for at least one week and become aware of the quality and quantity of food you are choosing.

− 20 −

Charts

The Dirty Dozen™ refers to the fruits and vegetables that are highest in pesticides and should always be purchased organic. The Clean 15™ refers to the fruits and vegetables lowest in pesticides that can be purchased conventionally. For more information: www.ewg.org

The Dirty Dozen and the Clean Fifteen Chart

Dirty Dozen™	Clean 15™
Apples	Asparagus
Celery	Avocados
Cherry Tomatoes	Cabbage
Cucumbers	Cantaloupe
Grapes	Sweet Corn
Hot Peppers	Egg Plant
Nectarines - Imported	Grapefruit
Peaches	Kiwi
Potatoes	Mangos
Spinach	Mushrooms
Strawberries	Onions
Sweet Bell Peppers	Papayas
Kale / Collards +	Pineapples
Summer Squash +	Sweet Peas Frozen
	Sweet Potatoes

Where Do I Find My Protein?

Food	Amount	Protein (g)	Protein (g/100 cal)
Alfalfa seeds, sprouted	1 cup	4	
Mung beans, sprouted	1 cup	3.0	
Peas, mature seeds sprouted	1 cup	8.8	
Lentils, sprouted	1 cup	9	
Radish seeds, sprouted	1 cup	3.8	
Garlic	1 clove	6.4	
Onions	1 med. 1 cup chopped	0.9	
Mushrooms, brown or Crimini raw	14 grams	2.5	
Lentils cooked	1 cup	18	7.8
Mung beans, cooked	1 cup	14	
Black beans, cooked	1 cup	15	6.7
Kidney beans, cooked	1 cup	13	6.4
Chickpeas, cooked	1 cup	12	4.2
Pinto beans, cooked	1 cup	12	5.7
Black-eyed, cooked	1 cup	11	6.2
Lima beans, cooked	1 cup	10	5.7
Veggie baked beans	1 cup	12	5.0
Green beans	1 cup	1.8	
Squash	1 cup cubes	1.4	
Cabbage, red	1 cup shredded	1.4	
Collards	1 cup chopped	2.5	
Cilantro	1 cup	2.1	
Quinoa	3 1/2 oz.	13.1	
Spaghetti, cooked	1 cup	8	3.7
Brown rice, cooked	1 cup	5	2.1
Wild rice	1 cup	14.7	
Millet	3 1/2 oz.	11.0	
Oats	3 1/2 oz.	13	
Buckwheat	3 1/2 oz.	13.3	
Amaranth	3 1/2 oz.	14.5	
Spelt	3 1/2 oz.	15	
Flaxseeds (whole)	1 tbsp.	2	

Where Do I Find My Protein?

Food	Amount	Protein (g)	Protein (g/100 cal)
Almonds	3 1/2 oz.	19	
Walnuts	3 1/2 oz.	15	
Sesame seeds	3 1/2 oz.	19	
Sunflower seeds	3 1/2 oz.	24	
Cashews	1/4 cup	5	2.7
Peanut butter	2 tbsp.	8	4.3
Almond butter	2 tbsp.	5	2.4
Broccoli	1 cup	4	6.8
Spinach, cooked	1 cup	2.9	
Lettuce	1 medium head	4.9	
Kale	3 1/2 oz.	4	
Brussels sprouts	3 1/2 oz.	5	
Parsley	3 1/2 oz.	4	
Potato, baked	1 med (6 oz.)	4	2.7
Sweet potato	1 med. 5"	1.6	
Tempeh (fermented soybean)	3 1/2 oz.	18	
Miso	3 1/2 oz.	12	
Nori	1 sheet	1.3	
Chlorella	100 grams	55	
Quinoa bread	2 slices	7	
Ezekiel 4.9 whole grain	1 slice	4	
Ezekiel 4.9 sprouted whole grain tortilla	1 tortilla	6	
Sourdough bread	3 1/2 oz.	10	
All fruits	3 1/2 oz.	1–2	
Durian fruit	1 cup	1.5	
Tomatoes, red	1 med	0.9	
Tomatoes, orange	1 fruit	1.2	
Tomatoes, sundried	1 cup	14.1	
Dates, Deglet Noor	1 med.	2.5	
Dates, Medjool	1 med, pitted	1.8	
Raisons, seedless	1 cup pkgd	3.1	

FOOTNOTES

1. • http://www.preventcancer.com/consumers/general/ hormones_meat.htm
   • http://healthychild.org/blog/comments/hormonal_milk_and _meat_ a_dangerous_public_health_risk/#ixzz1lcBSX3UZ
2. *Encyclopedia of Nutritional Supplements*, Michael T. Murray, N.D, ©1996 Michael T. Murray.
3. *Health by Purification*, Peter Jentschura and Josef Lohkamper, ©Verlag Peter Jentschura 1998.
4. *The Cellulite Solution*, Howard Murad, M.D.©2005 by Howard Murad, M.D.
5. *Cracking the Metabolic Code*, James B. LaValle, R.Ph., C.C.N., N.D., ©2004 by James B. LaValle, R.Ph.,C.C.N.,N.D.
6. *The Cellulite Solution*, Howard Murad, M.D.©2005 by Howard Murad, M.D.
7. *The pH Miracle for Weight Loss*, Robert O. Young, PhD, ©2005 by Hikari Holdings, LLC.
8. *Food & Mood, The Complete Guide to Eating Well and Feeling Your Best*, Elizabeth Somer, M.A., R.D. ©1995, 1999 by Elizabeth Somer.
9. *Encyclopedia of Nutritional Supplements*, Michael T. Murray, N.D, page 176, ©1996 Michael T. Murray.
10. *Health by Purification*, Peter Jentschura and Josef Lohkamper, ©Verlag Peter Jentschura 1998.
11. *Sexy Hormones*, Lorna R.Vanderhaeghe MS, Alvin Pettle, MD, ©2007 Lorna R. Vanderhaeghe M.S.and Alvin Pettle, M.D.
12. *Nutritional Pathology*, Stephney Whillier, ©1999 Stephney, Willier.
13. *YinSights, A Journey into the Philosophy & Practice of Yin Yoga*, Bernie Clark, © 2007 by Bernie Clark.
14. Rossi AB, Vergnanini AL (July 2000). "Cellulite: a review." *J Eur Acad Dermatol Venereol* 14 (4): 251–62. doi:10.1046/j.1468-3083.2000.00016.x.
15. http://www.drhoffman.com/page.cfm/183.
16. http://www.livestrong.com/article/16099-foods-reduce-estrogen- dominance/
17. http://envirocancer.cornell.edu/factsheet/general/fs10.estrogen.cfm

REFERENCES

Encyclopedia of Nutritional Supplements, Michael T. Murray, N.D, ©1996 Michael T. Murray.

Health by Purification, Peter Jentschura and Josef Lohkamper, ©Verlag Peter Jentschura 1998.

Cracking the Metabolic Code, James B. LaValle, R.Ph., C.C.N., N.D., ©2004 by James B. LaValle, R.Ph.,C.C.N.,N.D.

The Cellulite Solution, Howard Murad, M.D.©2005 by Howard Murad, M.D.

Your Right To Be Beautiful, The Miracle of Raw Foods, Tonya Zavasta, ©2003 by Antonina Zavastitsa.

Sexy Hormones, Lorna R. Vanderhaeghe MS, Alvin Pettle, MD, ©2007 Lorna R. Vanderhaeghe M.S. and Alvin Pettle, M.D.

Nutritional Pathology, Stephney Whillier, ©1999 Stephney, Willier.

The pH Miracle for Weight Loss, Robert O. Young, PhD, ©2005 by Hikari Holdings, LLC.

Food & Mood, The Complete Guide to Eating Well and Feeling Your Best, Detoxification, Linda Page, N.D., Ph.D. 1999-2002 by Traditional Wisdom, Inc.

Get It Ripe, Jae Steele 2008 Jae Steele.

The Complete Natural Medicine Guide to Woman's Health, Dr. Sat Dharam Kaur, ND, Dr. Mary Danylak-Arhanic, MD., Dr. Carolyn Dean, ND, MD, ©Sat Dharam Daur, Mary Danylak-Arhanic and Carolyn Dean, 2005.

RECIPE REFERENCES

Varicose Vein Tonic, pg. 134 — From *Detoxification,* by Linda Page, N.D., Ph.D. © 1999-2002 by Traditional Wisdom, Inc.

Coconut Cauliflower Stew, pg. 156 — Original recipe from the *Get it Ripe Cookbook* by Jae Steele © 2008 by Jae Steele. Modified into a low fat version

Spouted Mung Bean Patties, pg. 159 — Original recipe from *Simrit Gill*

Artichoke Paella, pg. 160 — Recipe from *The Starch Solution,* John A. McDougall, MD.

Energy Bars, pg. 162 — Modified from: http://www.happyhealthylonglife.com/happy_healthy_long_life/chia_bars.h tml

Raw Blueberry Pie, pg. 164 — Original recipe from *therawbuzz.com*

About the Author

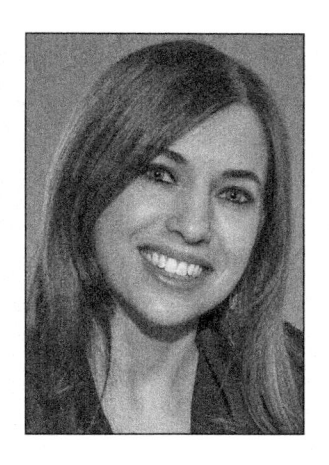

Ara Wiseman RHN, ROHP, RNCP, is a leading nutrition expert, anti-aging specialist, author, teacher, lecturer and yoga instructor. She has written and published three books; *Feed Your Body Feed Your Soul*, *The Healing Option* and *A Smoother You*. She is also the creator of Smart Cacao Inc., a boutique line of dark, raw, organic chocolate.

CPSIA information can be obtained
at www.ICGtesting.com
Printed in the USA
LVOW04s1120220616
493572LV00016B/64/P